Walking with GOD

Walking with GOD

THE 40-DAY FITNESS PROGRAM AND BIBLICAL JOURNEY

Anna Fitch Courie

morehouse PUBLISHING

Morehouse Publishing
19 East 34th Street
New York, NY 10016

Morehouse Publishing is an imprint of Church Publishing Incorporated.

Cover design by David Baldeosingh Rotstein
Typeset by Andrew Berry

Library of Congress Cataloging-in-Publication Data

Names: Fitch Courie, Anna author
Title: Walking with God : the 40-day fitness program and Biblical journey / Anna Fitch Courie.
Description: New York, NY : Morehouse Publishing, [2025]
Identifiers: LCCN 2024034364 | ISBN 9781640657823 ebook | ISBN 9781640657816 paperback
Subjects: LCSH: Health—Religious aspects—Christianity | Spiritual life—Christianity | Walking—Religious aspects—Christianity
Classification: LCC BT732 .F585 2025 | DDC 261.8/321—dc23/eng /20241015
LC record available at https://lccn.loc.gov/2024034364

This book is dedicated to my husband, Treb, who has been the best of companions on my own journey.

Contents

Introduction 1

PART I

TREKKING THROUGH THE OLD TESTAMENT

Day 1 Scaling the Tower of Babel 15

Day 2 Migrating with Abraham 21

Day 3 Jacob's Great Escape 25

Day 4 The Exodus to Freedom 31

Day 5 Crossing the Jordan 37

Day 6 The Queen of Sheba's Quest 41

Day 7 Ruth Relocates to Bethlehem 47

Day 8 Climbing Mount Horeb 53

Day 9 A Pilgrimage to Healing 59

Day 10 A Return from Exile 65

PART II

EXPLORING THE NEW TESTAMENT

Day 11	The Magi Go East	73
Day 12	The Flight into Egypt	77
Day 13	The Traveling Preacher	83
Day 14	On the Mountain with Jesus	89
Day 15	Stepping into the Healing Pools	97
Day 16	Crossing the Stormy Sea	103
Day 17	The Journey from Bethlehem to Jerusalem	107
Day 18	The Disciples Venture Out	113
Day 19	Resting at the Well	119
Day 20	The Way of the Cross	125

PART III

TRAVELING WITH THE APOSTLES

Day 21	The Road to Damascus	133
Day 22	Heading Back to Emmaus	139
Day 23	Paul's First Missionary Trip	145
Day 24	Coming to Corinth	151
Day 25	Preaching in Philippi	155
Day 26	Answering God's Call	161

Day 27 All Roads Lead to Rome 167
Day 28 Spreading the Word 173
Day 29 A Voyage to Crete 179
Day 30 On a Path to Wholeness 185

PART IV

WALKING WITH . . .

Day 31 Uncertainty 193
Day 32 Trauma 197
Day 33 Fear 203
Day 34 Worry 209
Day 35 The Unknown 213
Day 36 Doubt 217
Day 37 Anxiety 221
Day 38 Faith 227
Day 39 Revelation 233
Day 40 Wisdom 237

Afterword 241

Introduction

And Moses swore on that day, saying, "Surely the land on which your foot has trodden shall be an inheritance for you and your children for ever, because you have wholeheartedly followed the Lord *my God."*

—Joshua 14:9

When I started writing *Walking with God,* the world was in the midst of a quarantine due to COVID-19. I had been writing about Brother Lawrence, a fifteenth-century monk known for writing *Practice of the Presence of God,* and I was mulling over ways that I could find the extraordinary of God in the ordinariness of being stuck at home.

While there was nothing ordinary about a global pandemic, there was something missing in my life. I wanted to experience the joy of simple things, like making an omelet for breakfast—a point Br. Lawrence makes in his book. I yearned to find meaning in the everydayness, in the moments that we often overlook in our search for the extraordinary. After all, as the Bible shows us time and time again, extraordinary journeys often begin with the mundane. It involves common people like you and me: fathers, mothers, fishermen, tax collectors—many of whom do not start out as heros, but as ordinary men and women seeking God.

Walking with God is an exploration of these journeys and what God teaches us on those routes. If you are familiar with my previous *Christ Walk* books and the methodology of praying and walking on a journey with God, then you'll find a familiar cadence within these pages. I still call you to walk those miles physically (or run, swim, bike, exercise, volunteer, pray—whatever floats your boat), but I also want to explore what was going on in these journeys, what they mean today, and how those journeys can transform you as an individual.

Over the years of the *Christ Walk* program, I usually received two opposite yet equally extreme responses: Some wanted more prayer and reflection in their *Christ Walk,* while others wanted more activity. It is very much like having Mary and Martha write Amazon reviews! As a natural Martha myself, I enjoy the activity of spiritual movement. I am at heart a "do-er" and struggle with the "be-er" part of the Mary/Martha dichotomy. Consequently, I am actually trying to stretch myself with this book and explore the more spiritual and prayerful aspects of the journeys in the Bible like Mary would. I invite you to do the same over the next forty days because journeys are as spiritual as they are physical.

As I reflected on the dozens of journeys taken by my biblical forebears, I was reminded that my spiritual struggles are not unique. They've been experienced by millions of people in the past and will certainly be experienced by countless people in the future. The Bible has collected these journeys and experiences and recorded them, so we know we are not alone. God is with us.

I am a hands-on person; I need to touch and feel things to digest and understand the knowledge and experience derived from the event. Taking the steps on these different journeys lets me do that, and I think you will benefit from doing the same. As you will see, walking will become a physical manifestation to your commitment to your faith.

When I pray when I walk, each step represents a word in my prayer that I offer up to God. Lately, those words seem to represent a number of emotions that I am processing. Perhaps you feel these things too. With each step on my walk these days, I step and pray: "I am anxious," "I am scared," "I am tired, or "I am hopeless."

With every health hurdle, I have found similar words pouring forth in my prayer walk as I breathe out a phrase that has been resting on my mind. As I take each step, I imagine handing the word weighing on my mind to God (God is, after all, the Word of Words). And as I continue each daily walk or run or prayer, I begin to examine these words.

I am anxious because of the unknown. Times right now are beyond our control. I am unsure of the future. Sometimes I feel that I don't have as much "busyness" to keep me occupied, and my natural inclination to be anxious creeps forward into my frontal lobe. Are these feelings and thoughts that you have had as well?

I am tired. All these feelings are exhausting. All the news is overwhelming. The work that has been going on for me has been intense. I feel that the goings-on of the world is keeping me from the prayer life that keeps me centered. Are you tired as well? Do you also feel that when you catch your breath with one thing, something else happens? Do you ever feel that something else is thrust in your arms before you have that chance to rest? I feel this way.

These feelings are common. You aren't alone. These feelings aren't even unique. People can feel them when they are faced with illness, loss, abuse, trauma, moral injury, divorce, death, job loss, and many, many other human experiences. It's important to process these feelings, but how?

I walk.

I invite you to do the same.

What is *Walking with God?* This book is a spiritual fitness program. It is designed to improve your mind, body, and spiritual health. By pairing daily meditations with the stories of biblical journeys, you will be able to set a fitness goal. *Walking with God* uses the *Christ Walk* method to engage in a physical mileage goal while meditating on what God is teaching us in the journeys that make up the Bible. In many ways, this book seeks to encourage physical action while you process your own spiritual journey that is often associated with being out of balance in mind, body, or spirit.

Walking with God is also a personal reflection on my pursuit of spiritually and physically healthy life. After more than twenty years (!) of *Christ Walk,* I've found that people enjoy having a book as a companion when they go on journeys. The book in your hands is a manual/journal for you to have an interactive experience, and by the end of the forty days, it will be as much your book as it is mine.

Walking with God is designed for individuals or groups. It is designed to be used and reused because our walk with God should never end. There is always another journey. My hope for you is that these forty days transform you and encourage you to pursue new journeys and set new goals.

The Bible is filled with stories about journeys. God was using physical bodies for generations to transform the world. I would like for us to reclaim that relationship with our physical bodies and express our faith not only with our lips but also with our lives, fitness, health, cooking, care, and prayer. I am filled with awe that Christianity spread during a time when there were no cars, or trucks, or trains, or airplanes to get our prophets and disciples to the place where they wanted to spread the Word. There is a reason God gave us feet! We have feet to walk, run, jump, and skip through our lives. Our feet are to be used to care for the temple God created within each of us.

When I have struggled with how to live my life, I have always felt that God was there to help me and provide me with strength and guidance. I believe that the Bible is filled with instruction on how to seek from God the strength, guidance, and direction we need in all aspects of our personal well-being. I believe that God is foundational to a healthy life.

Each day follows a structured methodology: Read, Reflect, and Respond. There will be a Bible passage related to a specific journey in the Bible, my meditation on that content and how it relates to your personal well-being and struggles inherent in life, and then questions for you to digest the content from your own personal perspective. I also offer a modern-day interactive approach to fitness, suggesting apps and resources that can enrich your daily walk.

I encourage you to couple this process with a physical goal of running, walking, swimming, hiking, yoga, or whatever physical activity that will engage you with caring for your physical well-being. Some days may be more focused on the body and other days may be more centered on your spirit. All of these days will help you on your journey to a healthier you!

If you are physically unable to walk, I ask that you look at your life in ways that you can change it and improve it. Everyone has things that they can do to make their life healthier. Perhaps your goal will be to study something new on your journey or pray with more discipline or focus on changing your nutritional habits. If you cannot physically exercise, discuss with your health care provider on some options that you are willing to do to change. There is a place in this journey for everyone. We may need to be creative on the method that the journey is completed. I ask that you pray through those chapters that are not applicable to you and really focus on the ones that speak to your personal experience. I have tried to write to many different perspectives and needs. I am aware that this book will not work for everyone, but if you cannot make the journey on your own, consider how you can help others on their journey. Keep an open mind and again, consider, "What can I do to change?"

So how do we make a healthy body? We take care of it. We exercise it, we feed it, we nurture it, and we rest it. Scientifically, the best exercise that most people keep up with is walking. Most of the stories and journeys in the Bible were done by foot. Consequently, as you begin this journey with me, I am going to ask you to pick a walking goal to focus on during the next forty days. There are different walking goals depending on your fitness level. Some people have walked the *Via Dolorosa* (Jesus's journey through Jerusalem to His crucifixion, one of my favorite routes), others walked Jesus's birth and death (the distance between Bethlehem and Jerusalem), while others have walked Paul's missionary journeys. Of course, you may choose to set your own goal! It is up to you. But as we physically walk through our *Walking with God* journey, it will help to focus you on your spiritual goals as well.

As a reminder, some of the distances I include are estimates. Some are lost to antiquity. Some distances were estimated using a ruler and map grid, and others were calculated with Google Maps. I take full responsibility in any inaccuracies and beg your forgiveness if you may find any.

Some of these routes were chosen because they touched a very special part of me for different reasons. These biblical journeys represent different themes to me, and I will share with you how they became a part of my journey.

The second year I did *Christ Walk*, I learned that the journey was a lot more fun when we did it with teams. I see no reason why the same does not apply to *Walking with God*. The teams provided a support system to get each of us through our different strengths and weaknesses on our routes.

There may be another route that speaks more deeply to you than these favorites of mine, and I encourage you to find that route and journey it. The point is to get up and get moving and explore these different journeys in the Bible and see how they will change you. The journey cannot get started if you are sitting down.

Each day, there will be a place for you to fill in your steps/distance, your activity, your feelings for the day, and your spiritual thought for the day. Do not rush to finish the book. This book is designed to be read one chapter a day and as a journal to help you on your way and improve your *spiritual and physical* experience. If at any time you need to change your goals, feel free to do so. Life is a journey with many bumps! The challenge is that you continue to have faith to continue on the journey, even if it is in a different way than the one in which you started.

So, how do we measure the steps we took, the distance we traveled? I recommend the purchase of a fitness tracker, which can be worn on your wrist or clothing, and will track the number of steps/miles traveled each day. Recommendations from the experts encourage every individual to take 10,000 steps a day for heart health. You may need to work up to this level of activity, and perhaps this will be one of your goals. Just 2,000 more steps a day in your life can make a huge difference in your well-being. If 10,000 steps is overwhelming, start with your average and set a goal to go just a little bit farther each day. Roughly 2,000 to 2,500 steps equal a mile. For the purpose of this program, we generally give one mile for every 2,000 steps.

If you want to use another form of exercise other than walking (biking, swimming, aerobics, dance, etc.), you may do so. It takes about fifteen minutes to walk a mile, so every 15-minute block of exercise can be calculated as a mile. The important thing is to choose an activity that you enjoy and do it. The purpose is to get out there and move, to think about every step you take as walking with God. This is your walk and your journey—focus on quality steps with God and the rest will come together! Your job is to give it your best shot with all your heart.

In *Walking with God,* my goal for you is to set mind, body, and spirit goals that will help you focus on God. Our bodies are temples of the Holy Spirit. I believe that God works through each of us. I believe that we are the arms and feet and lips of the Church in the world and just like any other piece of valuable equipment, we need to take care of it. We are all different. We are all different shapes and sizes and all different levels of health, wellness, and physical capability, but we all have a bit of Christ within us. Therefore, we should take care of that temple that God has given us. A healthy body can do more for others and share Christ's love within us in whatever capacity we are called to serve.

As I've said before, these are my thoughts, feelings, beliefs, and experiences. I will use a lot of "I" statements since my experiences shaped my theological beliefs on the topic of trauma, health, wellness, and the path to healing. If these thoughts and feelings and beliefs do not resonate with your own experience, that is okay. All of our experiences collectively are shaping the Christian community's testament to God in the world. It is all good when it is done for the love of Christ. I hope that these meditations help you along on your journey and that you feel free to make it your own.

THOUGHTS TO PONDER

1. What is my goal?
2. How do I feel about my goal? Is it reasonable/attainable/realistic? If not, how can I make it something that I will stick with the next forty days?
3. Who can I reach out to to help me on my journey?
4. What do you think about the passage from Joshua 14:9 in relationship to your own journey?

My physical goal for *Walking with God* the next forty days is:

____

____

____

My spiritual goal for *Walking with God* the next forty days is:

____

____

____

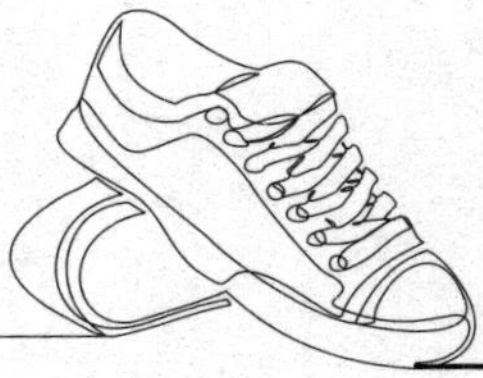

Part

1

Trekking through the Old Testament

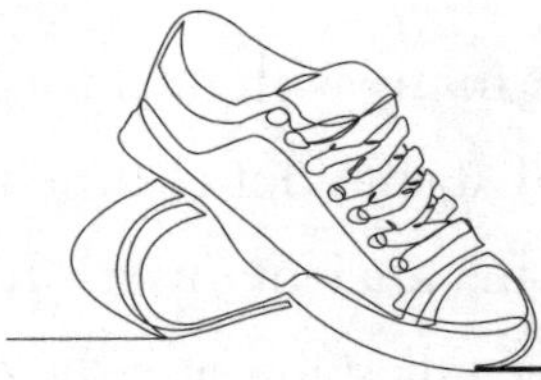

Day 1

Scaling the Tower of Babel

So the Lord scattered them abroad from there over the face of all the earth, and they left off building the city. Therefore it was called Babel, because there the Lord confused the language of all the earth; and from there the Lord scattered them abroad over the face of all the earth.

—Genesis 11:8–9

THE TOWER OF BABEL: Height unknown
TALLEST TOWER IN THE WORLD: Tokyo Sky Tree, Tokyo, Japan, 2,080 feet

In 2002, while I was living in Germany with my husband, who was an Army JAG officer, I spent a lot of time traveling throughout Europe and climbing ancient towers. It was almost like a rite of passage to find the tallest tower in the town or city we were visiting and journey up to the top. From the pinnacle of the Zugspitze, the Tower of Pisa, the bell towers of Tuscany, or the dome of St. Paul's, we were able to glimpse the most magnificent views throughout Europe.

We have continued this beloved tradition wherever we have lived in the world. Treb and I have been to the Seattle Space Needle, the Sears Tower, and the Empire State Building. One of my personal favorites, however, is far from America. It's the Tokyo Tower. From the top of this incredible landmark, we

WHAT'S IN YOUR JOURNEY BACKPACK?

Item 1: I use a Fitbit watch religiously (no pun intended) to track my miles. It's useful to have a digital fitness tracker (Fitbit, Apple Watch, Garmin, Smart Band, Amazfit) connected to your phone to track how far you walk and move on your daily journey. But if you feel this is an expensive investment, you can use a pedometer, which is more affordable, and attach it to your pants/belt to track your miles manually.

were able to see the city stretching on and on and the thousands and thousands of people bustling about below.

As I stood atop the Tokyo Tower, I was reminded of the story of the Tower of Babel. In the story, the people built a tower to reach the heavens. Some theologians think this is supposed to represent the hubris of the people. Others have reflected that it represents our human desire to be like God. Either way, God found it fit to teach the people of Babel a lesson by making them speak in different languages. Consequently, the tower crumbled, symbolizing that our humanity's efforts to be like God is futile.

There's nothing more humbling than trying to communicate with someone who does not speak the same language as you. I've learned this time and time again, especially as an English-speaking American traveler and also as a person who lost her hearing when she was young. In fact, when I hear different languages (sometimes even my spoken English!), it often sounds like babble—a word which happens to derive from Babel. The conflict inherent in different communication patterns defines our struggles as humans to find that critical point of where we find meaning together as individuals. Speaking in different languages forces us to take the time to understand one another. It forces us to be compassionate and patient and caring. While God understands all our languages, it is only through work that we are able to understand one another.

God's command for us to love our neighbor threads its way all throughout the Bible. This command weaves it through all of Jesus's teachings on how we interact with other people. The Tower of Babel isn't so much a story of God's punishment but a reminder of how hard it is to work toward understanding one another in spite of our many, many differences. Our personal pride, sovereignty, and self-assurance crumbles when we seek to understand one another. When we truly seek understanding, we realize we are nothing without God.

THOUGHTS TO PONDER

1. Have you ever listened to the Bible in another language? If not, try it. It's incredibly frustrating. You may take for granted your understanding of the Word of God until you try to understand it in a language that is not your own.
2. What is something you do not understand about another person, or something they believe? Why does it frustrate you?
3. What are ways that you've learned to develop patience and kindness for another person whose beliefs are not your own?

Steps taken: ____________ Miles journeyed: ____________

Exercise chosen: ____________________________________

Something I thought about:

____

____

____

____

Something I need to pray about:

____

____

____

____

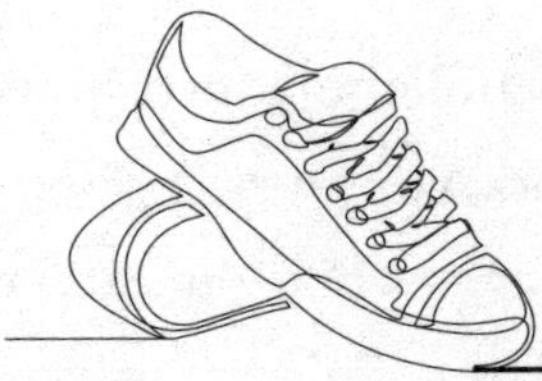

Day 2

Migrating with Abraham

Now the LORD said to Abram, "Go from your country and your kindred and your father's house to the land that I will show you. I will make of you a great nation, and I will bless you, and make your name great, so that you will be a blessing.

So Abram went, as the LORD had told him; and Lot went with him. Abram was seventy-five years old when he departed from Haran. Abram took his wife Sarai and his brother's son Lot, and all the possessions that they had gathered, and the persons whom they had acquired in Haran; and they set forth to go to the land of Canaan.

—Genesis 12:1–2, 4–5

UR TO ISRAEL: 792 miles (estimated)

Life is hard. It's been hard for millennia, ever since, in fact, the dawn of humankind. However, I often find that we can make sense of our struggles and our sufferings when we turn to God and trust in Him. This is illustrated in the story of Abraham, whom God calls to leave all he knows behind and journey to a new and unknown land.

Imagine if God called you to leave your home and to migrate—on foot!—to a place that was strange to you. How would you feel? How would you react? I know I would push back and ask countless questions and voice all kinds of doubts. But Abraham isn't called our forefather for nothing. He trusted in God and followed God's call for his life. He heard, prayed, and followed the path God had made for him. Abraham

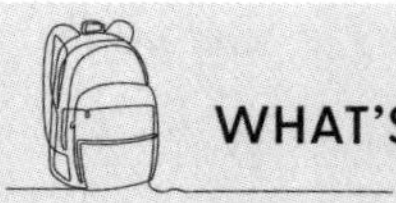

WHAT'S IN YOUR JOURNEY BACKPACK?

Item #2: Every walk I take includes listening to the *Pray as You Go* podcast. Each day includes a beautiful choral piece, a reading from the daily lectionary, and a short reflection that encourages you to respond to God's Word on your walk. Find a spiritually enriching podcast that works for you and listen to it as you journey. I promise it will make walking easier and more rewarding!

prostrated himself before the Lord and put all of himself as an offering to God.

We are told in the Psalms that the psalmists, like Abraham, prostrate themselves in the sight of the Lord. This physical bowing down is a surrender to God, their way of saying, "Here I am, Lord. Here is my suffering. Here is my pain. I cannot do this on my own." We can learn something from Abraham and the psalmists. They do not get stuck in the past, in their pain. They see a means to push forward. They see a future and hope.

Do you give all of yourself, all of your suffering, all of your pain to God? Or do you nurture it, hold on to it, stroke it, and wear it like armor? Abraham's story is one of surrender before God, to something—or rather, Someone—that is greater than himself. What would happen if you did the same?

THOUGHTS TO PONDER

1. Are you holding on to your pain and suffering like a weapon?
2. Is part of your journey calling you to let go of something?
3. Is God asking you to come along for a long trip and to trust in Him?

Steps taken: ____________ Miles journeyed: ____________

Exercise chosen: ________________________________

Something I thought about:

____

____

____

____

Something I need to pray about:

____

____

____

____

Day

3

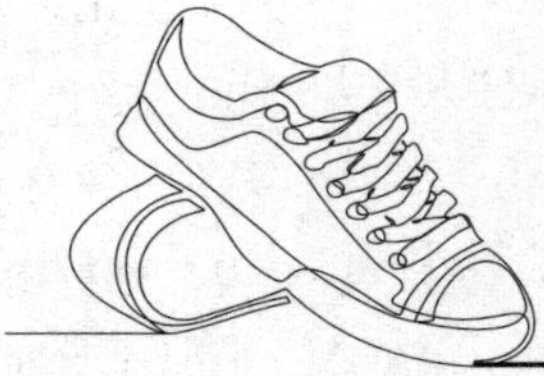

Jacob's Great Escape

The same night he got up and took his two wives, his two maids, and his eleven children, and crossed the ford of the Jabbok. He took them and sent them across the stream, and likewise everything that he had. Jacob was left alone; and a man wrestled with him until daybreak. When the man saw that he did not prevail against Jacob, he struck him on the hip socket; and Jacob's hip was put out of joint as he wrestled with him.

Then the man said, "You shall no longer be called Jacob, but Israel, for you have striven with God and with humans, and have prevailed."

—Genesis 32:22–25, 28

BETHEL TO HARAN: 400 miles
BETHEL TO PENIEL: 30 miles

The story of Jacob wrestling with God is one with which many Christians are familiar. I know that when I am struggling, it feels as though I am wrestling with God myself. I see myself in Jacob's shoes—or sandals!—and I find my fallible human will struggling against God's perfect one. And even though I know intellectually that God's way is better than my own feeble attempts to control my life, still I wrestle. I demand that God conform to my will and bless my desires and plans, much like Jacob.

In this story, Jacob has gone on a journey to escape his brother, Esau, for he was afraid that Esau would kill him for having tricked him out of his birthright. Along the way, Jacob ends up in the camp of his uncle Laban and falls in love with Laban's daughter Rachel. In order to earn the right to marry Rachel, Jacob agrees to work for Laban for seven years. But,

WHAT'S IN YOUR JOURNEY BACKPACK?

Item #3: Get shoes that fit comfortably. If you are new to physical fitness, it's worth going to a running shoe store or another specialty store to be properly fitted for shoes. There's nothing worse than starting out on a journey and going off course because of blisters or foot pain. Get good shoes.

when the seven years is complete, Jacob is tricked into marrying Laban's older daughter, Leah. Jacob is enraged but ultimately agrees to work for Laban for another seven years to marry his one, true love.

After serving Laban for so long, Jacob is called back to Canaan, and he decides to return home. On his way back to Canaan, an angel of the Lord appears before Jacob, and they wrestle. Jacob's determination helps him win the match, and the angel in turn blesses him. Jacob ultimately comes to the conclusion he was wrestling with God and names the place of this event "Peniel," meaning, "I saw God face-to-face and yet my life was spared."

Jacob's journey to find Rachel was a long one. It was likely over four hundred miles to return to the land of Abraham. There is a part of me that wonders if this journey was so long because Jacob was still internally working out his issues with Esau. Perhaps he needed the times to confront his fears and worries. The shorter journey—Bethel to Peniel is roughly thirty miles long—is one where God is pushing Jacob back home. And Jacob needs God's blessing to deal with his worry and fear in meeting with Esau.

But what if Jacob had wrestled the angel of the Lord at the beginning of his journey? What if his journey had first started with God and his relationship with Esau had been healed earlier? I think that it would have saved Jacob a lot of grief and trouble. But even though Jacob struggled and suffered during this long and arduous journey, many good things came of it.

For instance, he met Rachel and Leah, who would give birth to his children, the progenitors of the twelve tribes of Israel. Therefore, every moment of the journey Jacob was growing and learning about grace, mercy, and patience. Is the better road the shorter one or the longer one?

I know that while some journeys would be a lot easier if we turn to God first, I also know that sometimes the painful and difficult and hard journeys we take are teaching us things along the way. No matter how traumatic your experiences may be, they are shaping you and teaching you as a part of that journey.

When we look at the science of posttraumatic growth,[*] we find evidence that learning from, exploring, and sharing the trauma opens paths for new meaning, deeper personal relationships, spiritual and existential growth, an appreciation for life, and personal strength.[†]

As an advocate for mental health and wellness, I've often struggled that I cannot take away the ills of the world. I wish nothing more than for people not to be inflicted with traumatic

---

* Tedeschi, Richard G., and Lawrence G. Calhoun. 2004. "A Clinical Approach to Posttraumatic Growth." In *Positive Psychology in Practice,* edited by P. Alex Linley and Stephen Joseph. John Wiley & Sons, Inc. https://doi.org/10.1002/9780470939338.ch25.

† If you have experienced trauma and are struggling, please seek help. Your life is sacred, and you have purpose and meaning in this world. You can reach out for help at the Suicide Prevention Lifeline 988 to talk to a trained counselor; seek a trusted priest/minister; or other trained clinician to help you.

experiences. But I cannot fix that. I cannot take away trauma. But I think if we face trauma, share it, hold it gently and carefully, and give it to God, we may be able to find an opportunity for growth, a development of new meaning, and a sense of purpose following the trauma. When you struggle, imagine God in that moment with you. Imagine seeing the face of God like Jacob and being blessed.

THOUGHTS TO PONDER

1. Are you struggling with something? Has it been a struggle for a long time or a short time?
2. What do you think the face of God looks like?
3. Do you think your experiences can help others face their own struggles? If so, how do you share that?

Steps taken: ____________ Miles journeyed: ____________

Exercise chosen: ______________________________

Something I thought about:

____

____

____

____

Something I need to pray about:

____

____

____

____

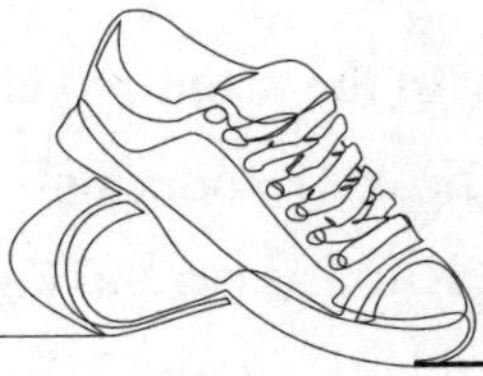

Day 4

The Exodus to Freedom

The Israelites journeyed from Rameses to Succoth, about six hundred thousand men on foot, besides children. A mixed crowd also went up with them, and livestock in great numbers, both flocks and herds.

The time that the Israelites had lived in Egypt was four hundred thirty years. At the end of four hundred thirty years, on that very day, all the companies of the Lord *went out from the land of Egypt.*

—Exodus 12:37–38, 40–41

RAMESES TO JERUSALEM: 462 Miles, 10 hours by car
RAMESES TO SUKKOTH: Unknown

The Jewish Exodus from Egypt to the promised land was not a journey for the faint of heart. Exodus tells us that the first leg of the journey was from Rameses to Sukkoth. My humble googling does not pop up Sukkoth on any map for me to trace, but ancient Rameses is thought to have been in the northeast corner of Egypt. I estimate (again with my trusty Google Maps app, a ruler, and some maps of the ancient world) that Rameses to Jerusalem is about 462 miles. I would guess that a group of six hundred thousand men plus women and children would not move very fast and that they probably did not make the trip all at the same time or at the same speed.

In fact, when we look at history, the migration of groups of people usually happens over a period of time. Regardless, if we take into consideration that the Israelites were likely better

WHAT'S IN YOUR JOURNEY BACKPACK?

Item #4: If you are going on a long distance journey or traversing difficult terrain, invest in hiking poles. I have a terrific pair of collapsable poles (easy for packing!) that I cannot live without when going hiking or walking. I have very poor balance from my hearing loss, so the poles provide me with extra reassurance. They will also increase your caloric burn by up to 20 percent.

at walking than we are today, I still will guess that the first stop in Sukkoth was likely about twenty miles away at most. Add in hunger, heat, grumpy children, and tired mamas, those twenty miles probably felt like forever and that was just the start of the 450-mile exodus. However, they made the journey anyway.

The people's minds (and hearts) were their biggest muscles. The Jews believed that God would be faithful to their covenant and deliver them from the slavery of Egypt. So, they walked. And walked. And walked. When they were tired or stumbled, they thought about God's promise and walked again. They used their minds and hearts to power their weary bodies to a place where they believed something better waited.

Do you think there is something better waiting for you? Is it hard or easy for you to see to end point? What do you think God's covenant means to you on your current journey? Are you using your mind and heart as much as you can to power you to where you want to be?

Journeys are hard. Sometimes we start on them not knowing how long they will be—much like the Israelites. We can take steps toward a goal and feel really good at first. The first leg of the journey usually has us really pumped and positive. However, there comes a point in every journey when the end seems elusive. The journey seems too long and too far. We get tired. The repetition seems boring. We cannot see the endgame, and we begin to doubt that the journey will even help us get to where we had planned.

I, for one, am really bad about seeing my destination. I often get caught up in the emotions of the present. I forget the wisdom of experience when I am under stress. My family and I once hiked the lava fields on the Big Island in Hawai'i. It was a tremendous effort heading out midafternoon toward the place on the mountain where lava oozes from earth's crust. We did great getting to the lava, and as the sun set, we experienced a once-in-a-lifetime display of God's glory.

As we headed back to town, we lit our headlamps to light our way. But the combination of scintillating light, the pitch dark, and the uneven rocky path beneath me triggered vertigo. We were two hours away from our car, and I wasn't sure I was going to make it. My head spun, I stumbled, and I was scared. My mind froze. I wasn't sure if I could make it or how long it would take and what it would entail for me to get home safely. So, I did the only thing I could do within my power. I prayed. And I held my husband's hand for stability and to ground me. And step by step, prayer by prayer, we made our way back.

The journey of the Israelites was similarly one of faith. They did not know how long the journey would be. They did not know where they would end up. In fact, they did not really know why they were even going on this journey beyond escaping the murderous pharaoh. It's likely that many did not even realize what a better life would look like.

Often in our personal journeys, the catalyst for us to take that first step toward change is "anything but this." We realize that change needs to be made in our lives, that we are a slave to something, and we desperately want freedom. That catalyst to change is a good thing. You need to hold on to the belief that things can get better when your journey becomes tough, long, boring, and may seem pointless.

In our Christian heritage, the crucifixion represents Christ's final sacrifice for our sins. His resurrection is a promise that God will make all things whole.* From birth, to death, to resurrection, Christ's journey is one of transformation and faith. His death is the catalyst that things cannot be the same. It's that "anything but this" moment in history that calls us all to change and be transformed and opened to the promise that wholeness is a part of God's love and promise for us.

The message from the journey of Exodus is to never stop walking. Never give up hope. Never give up faith. There is a promised land waiting for you at the end of your journey. So, just keep walking.

* Please note, God's time and our time is not the same thing.

THOUGHTS TO PONDER

1. Do you think there is something better waiting for you?
2. What do you think God's covenant means to you on your current journey?
3. Are you using your mind and heart as much as you can to power you to where you want to be?

Steps taken:__________ Miles journeyed:__________

Exercise chosen:______________________________

Something I thought about:

____

____

____

____

Something I need to pray about:

____

____

____

____

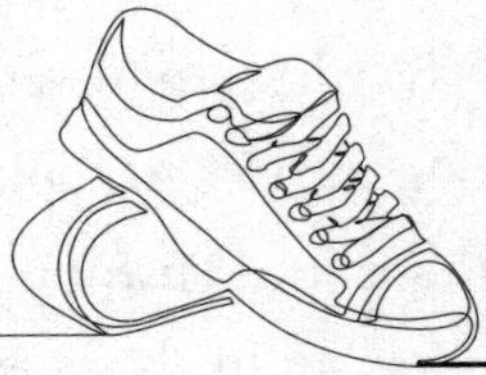

Day 5

Crossing the Jordan

The LORD was angry with me because of you, and he vowed that I should not cross the Jordan and that I should not enter the good land that the LORD your God is giving for your possession. For I am going to die in this land without crossing over the Jordan, but you are going to cross over to take possession of that good land. So be careful not to forget the covenant that the LORD your God made with you, and not to make for yourselves an idol in the form of anything that the LORD your God has forbidden you. For the LORD your God is a devouring fire, a jealous God.

—Deuteronomy 4:21–25

JORDAN RIVER LENGTH: 156 miles long
JORDAN RIVER WIDTH: About 15 miles at the widest part

The Israelites had to cross the river Jordan to get home. This river was a 156-mile-long barrier to their destination, with widths up to fifteen miles and rushing waters that flowed into the Dead Sea. The Jordan likely gave God's people pause.

God had promised the Israelites a home to call their own once they crossed the river. There was a promised land on the other side. All God asked them was to keep the covenant, to have faith, to trust Him in their crossing. God asks the same of us on our journeys. He assures us that there is a place for us to call home. Of course, this doesn't mean that there won't be

WHAT'S IN YOUR JOURNEY BACKPACK?

Item #5: The Journal app. I don't love journaling, but I do appreciate knowing where I was compared to where I am today. So, I use the Journal app on my iPhone to capture brief moments of faith and gratitude. These short snippets allow me to see my faith in action over time. The nice thing is you can journal on it as much or as little as you want. If you don't have an iPhone or prefer to use another app, there are plenty of other similar resources available online. Of course, a good, old-fashioned journal will also work.

pain or that people won't be left behind like Moses, who died before he reached his destination. It also doesn't mean there won't be suffering. However, God reminds us time and time again that through faith, a new home awaits, that a promise lies just beyond the river. In fact, on the other side, God is right there, patiently anticipating our coming. As we work through our fears and trepidations and shame, He waits lovingly for us as we make our journey. He knows that secretly we don't believe we can cross that river, that we are not worthy of that home, that we have sinned. But still, He is patient and loves us anyway.

Throughout scripture, throughout all these journeys, the one consistent thread is that God is faithful and keeps His covenant. God promises a home and a redeemer, and everywhere in scripture His promises are kept and fulfilled. God asks us to keep coming back to the covenant. And through Him, we can cross any river that stands as an obstacle before us. And we will never be able to fathom the glorious life that waits for us all.

THOUGHTS TO PONDER

1. Is there a river in your life that you are contemplating crossing?
2. What's it like? How does it make you feel?
3. Are there things you can do to prepare for a river crossing? Or does it simply take faith?

Steps taken: ___________ Miles journeyed: ___________

Exercise chosen: ___________________________________

Something I thought about:

____

____

____

____

Something I need to pray about:

____

____

____

____

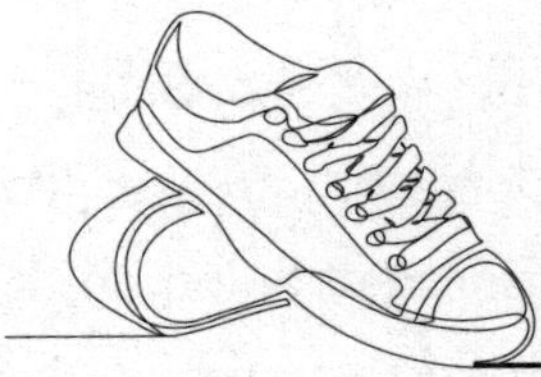

Day 6

The Queen of Sheba's Quest

When the queen of Sheba heard of the fame of Solomon (fame due to the name of the Lord*), she came to test him with hard questions. She came to Jerusalem with a very great retinue, with camels bearing spices, and very much gold, and precious stones; and when she came to Solomon, she told him all that was on her mind.*

When the queen of Sheba had observed all the wisdom of Solomon, the house that he had built, the food of his table, the seating of his officials, and the attendance of his servants, their clothing, his valets, and his burnt offerings that he offered at the house of the Lord, there was no more spirit in her.

—1 Kings 10:1–2, 4–5

SHEBA TO JERUSALEM: Roughly 683 miles

The Queen of Sheba traveled from Sheba (or Saba, which is thought to be in the modern-day area of Marib, Yemen) because she heard of the wisdom of Solomon. It was a very long journey. For context, Sheba to Jerusalem is very close to the distance from South Carolina to New York. This journey would have taken days to months to complete by foot, and a large caravan may have been required to carry everything a queen could possibly need on such a journey. They don't speak about it in the Bible, but it would not surprise me that people got sick or even died along the way. Journeys are not always safe or fun.

WHAT'S IN YOUR JOURNEY BACKPACK?

Item #6: Something sweet. I usually have a stash of something with a bit of sugar in my backpack. My current favorite is dark chocolate covered peanuts. The balance of sweet, salty, some protein, and fiber are just the thing you need when energy starts to flag. Likewise, sometimes you meet people on your journey that need a little something to pick them up. A bit of sweet, or a bit of a kind word, is often the thing they need too.

But the Queen of Sheba wanted to know of the wisdom of Solomon and his devotion to God. She wanted to understand how he built his houses, how he treated his servants, how he interacted with his officials, and how he worshipped God. She struggled to believe that Solomon could be a kind, wise, and compassionate leader without seeing it with her own eyes. I think it's incredibly appropriate that she did so. Learning itself is a journey—a dynamic journey of discovery. Learning takes practice, repetition, curiosity, a desire for things to be different, and a search for understanding for things we don't understand.

Often, we go on journeys to learn things from other people, to understand what others have discovered about the world, life, and often, tragedy. Learning from others creates a shared human experience that brings us closer together. In exchange for Solomon's wisdom, Sheba provided gold, spices, and other offerings. The Bible ultimately states that the exotic queen returned to her own lands. I like to think that she brought the wisdom of Solomon back with her and then implemented change in her own homeland.

When we share those lessons we've learned from our own troubles, we plant sacred spaces. Wisdom grows, and love and hope flourish. Those sacred spaces are spaces of communion. And where there are two or three people gathered, there is God. And that's how we build the Church. Every journey you take builds the Church because it provides you with the opportunity to spread love and wisdom. So, remember: searching for wisdom and knowledge is an important journey—one that requires the heart just as much as the body. It helps you grow, realize many important truths, and power through life's struggles.

THOUGHTS TO PONDER

1. What is an experience that you have had that could be shared in a sacred space?
2. Did you have to go on a journey to understand why this happened to you?
3. Do you think you grew from the experience?
4. How have you shared that with others?

Steps taken: ____________ Miles journeyed: ___________

Exercise chosen: ____________________________________

Something I thought about:

____

____

____

____

Something I need to pray about:

____

____

____

____

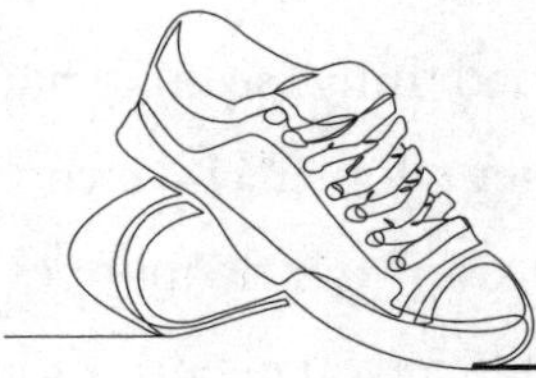

Day 7

Ruth Relocates to Bethlehem

But Ruth said, "Do not press me to leave you or to turn back from following you! Where you go, I will go; where you lodge, I will lodge; your people shall be my people, and your God my God. Where you die, I will die—there will I be buried. May the Lord *do thus and so to me, and more as well, if even death parts me from you!" When Naomi saw that she was determined to go with her, she said no more to her. So the two of them went on until they came to Bethlehem.*

—Ruth 1:16–19

JUDAH TO BETHLEHEM: About 30 miles

Have you ever wondered why bad things seem to happen to one person more than other people? Have you ever wondered why struggle and tragedy aren't a little more evenly distributed across the human race? Have you ever questioned why some people survive the greatest losses and still have faith?

I have. In fact, during a recent interview, I was asked to name someone I greatly admire as a hero or heroine. I drew a blank. No one came to mind that didn't seem trite or unimaginative, but what kept coming to mind were the traits I admired about multiple people.

I admire perseverance in the face of unimaginable tragedy. I admire grit. I admire steadfast faith. I admire people who show up on the worst days of someone's life, and I admire people who care more for individuals than their own well-being.

The account of Ruth and Naomi is a story of characteristics that I believe we should adopt, especially in the face of when bad things happen. Like all the stories of the Bible, Naomi and Ruth's teach us about the struggles many before us have experienced and how we too may respond in the face of repeated tragedies. Suffering, after all, is a part of the human condition, and it is how we respond individually and collectively that demonstrates our faith in response to trauma.

If we look to the story of Naomi, she is facing isolation, loss of her husband and her sons, and a lonely existence in which to live out her remaining years. She feels she has nothing left to offer. And yet, she urges her daughters-in-law to move on, to live their own lives, and to seek new relationships. She sees a future that is more than just loss.

Orpah and Ruth represent an almost Martha vs. Mary response to this situation. Neither response is wrong, but rather choices we can make when loss is a part of our family dynamic. Orpah seeks to move on. She takes Naomi's guidance to go back home after the death of her husband and seek new relationships, new beginnings. Orpah takes one path from her loss.

Ruth chooses to stay with Naomi. And in this choice, Ruth and Naomi travel together on to Bethlehem, where Boaz sees Ruth's faithfulness in caring for her mother-in-law. This journey brings Ruth and Boaz together, and their union later culminates in the birth of David, the direct ancestor of Jesus.

Ruth's choice to love and care for her widowed mother-in-law therefore paves a way for the coming of the savior of the world. Her life is a testament that there is always a future after

WHAT'S IN YOUR JOURNEY BACKPACK?

Item #7: *Forward Day by Day*. I need a daily practice that helps me remember God's presence in the mundane of every day. The small daily devotionals and readings produced by Forward Movement in *Forward Day by Day* are easy to stash in my journey backpack.

loss. Although it is easy to feel that good things can never occur after trauma, that is not true. Ruth's story tells us that hope is alive, that when bad things happen, we can decide how we respond. Will we respond with anger, fear, negativity? Or will we respond with love and compassion, like Ruth? Bitterness is easy. And while love is hard, it heals and restores and paves pathways of hope. Ruth's love for Naomi healed her, and it healed Ruth. And through Ruth's love, we have the family of Jesus. It might not take trauma and tragedy away from our memory, but love sure does make the journey bearable—and even beautiful.

THOUGHTS TO PONDER

1. Have you experienced trauma?
2. Have you or do you feel like you are at crossroads, a point of choice following your trauma?
3. Are there ways you can lean into love and relationships with your experience?
4. Have you felt where love from someone else has helped you with your trauma?

Steps taken: ___________ Miles journeyed: ___________

Exercise chosen: ________________________________

Something I thought about:

____

____

____

____

Something I need to pray about:

____

____

____

____

Day 8

Climbing Mount Horeb

But . . . neither . . . forget . . . how you once stood before the Lord your God at Horeb, when the Lord said to me, "Assemble the people for me, and I will let them hear my words, so that they may learn to fear me as long as they live on the earth, and may teach their children so"; you approached and stood at the foot of the mountain while the mountain was blazing up to the very heavens, shrouded in dark clouds. Then the Lord spoke to you out of the fire. You heard the sound of words but saw no form; there was only a voice. He declared to you his covenant, which he charged you to observe, that is, the ten commandments; and he wrote them on two stone tablets.

—Deuteronomy 4:9–13

MOUNT HOREB: 7,497 feet

The locations and topography of the Bible are significant. They allow us to understand the history and context of the world in which the people of God lived and give us insight into their struggles and their victories, their heartaches and their hopes. Imagine right now a significant event in your life—a wedding, the birth of a child, a traumatic accident, a death. You will often describe each event in the context of the environment in which it occurred. Your senses may then be triggered, and you will be able to describe things that you tasted, touched, heard, felt, or smelled in that moment. These experiences make that event real to you.

I find this description of Mount Horeb to be especially meaningful. On Mount Horeb, the commandments of God were handed to God's people. This was a landmark event. The Jewish people were no longer wandering and alone—they were *chosen.* They had a God. They were given rules that would assure their prosperity and happiness. Like the Israelites, we are entreated to be vigilant and constantly remember that pivotal moment on the mount. One of the most signifant commands God gave the Israelites prohibited idolatry. But idolatry was not limited to serving other gods. No, throughout scripture the people of God will understand that idols can be anything—one's self, food, money, stature, fame, looks, drugs, alcohol, among many others.

Go climb the height of Mount Horeb. It will be hard. It will take work. A *lot* of work. Keeping God's commandments, like making journeys, requires discipline. But when we are diligent, when we keep to the commandments and the call of God in our lives, it is then that we see God.

I have been struggling lately chasing a promotion. I feel it is deserved, that I earned it. It isn't about the money, but it's definitely a lot about what I think I am due and a whole heck of a lot about my ego. I've been putting my career and goals ahead of my faith, and you know what? I haven't been happy. It's robbed me of the joy that I have always had doing the work I do for the people I serve. Chasing this promotion has made me forget who I am. I have been chasing an idol, and I didn't realize it until I sat down and read this passage. As the words flowed, I realized that I am guilty of chasing idols instead of chasing God—of breaking God's command to not commit idolatry.

WHAT'S IN YOUR JOURNEY BACKPACK?

Item #8: A silver cross. I wear a silver cross around my neck. It was a gift from my mother and father. It is a talisman, if you will, something that I reach up and touch when I pray, or when I'm stressed, or afraid. It's a physical representation to remind me I am never alone on my journey, no matter how hard things may be.

On today's journey, I want to think about the height of Mount Horeb. I want to move as though it was a climb, a trek, a scramble to the top, because more than anything, more than any promotion, any money, and status, I want to see God. And that means, just like the first people of God, I need to be diligent. Disciplined. Focused. Keep working at the commandments, and I promise that everything else will fall into place.

THOUGHTS TO PONDER

1. What are the idols in your life?
2. Where are you struggling right now that is turning your focus from God to worldly things?
3. What is a tough climb with which you can challenge yourself as a reminder that discipline is hard and we must continually reorient ourselves to God?
4. What is something that will make you work harder for God?

Steps taken: __________ Miles journeyed: __________

Exercise chosen: ______________________________

Something I thought about:

____

____

____

____

Something I need to pray about:

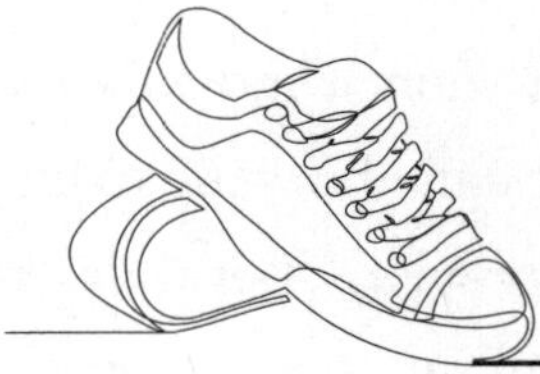

Day 9

A Pilgrimage to Healing

Naaman, commander of the army of the king of Aram, was a great man and in high favor with his master, because by him the Lord *had given victory to Aram. The man, though a mighty warrior, suffered from leprosy. Now the Arameans on one of their raids had taken a young girl captive from the land of Israel, and she served Naaman's wife. She said to her mistress, "If only my lord were with the prophet who is in Samaria! He would cure him of his leprosy."*

So Naaman came with his horses and chariots, and halted at the entrance of Elisha's house. Elisha sent a messenger to him, saying, "Go, wash in the Jordan seven times, and your flesh shall be restored and you shall be clean."

So he went down and immersed himself seven times in the Jordan, according to the word of the man of God; his flesh was restored like the flesh of a young boy, and he was clean.

—2 Kings 5:1–3, 9–10, 14

SYRIA TO SAMARIA: 280 miles

Have you ever been in a situation where you look to God and want God to wave a magic wand to fix your problems? Have you been ill and prayed, "Lord, just make it go away?" Have you ever been willing to try anything, do anything, go anywhere, desperately in search of relief, healing, succor?

I have. At the age of twelve, I lost my hearing to an autoimmune disease after contracting a viral infection. The medications the doctors put me on caused a lot of damage to my body, and I still have scars on my arms and legs. In fact, those medications that I was given in an attempt to preserve my hearing later resulted in a lymphoma diagnosis at the age of thirty-eight. It never fails to confound me that when we try to fix one thing, doing so may lead to another problem. My body, for me, has always been a source of frustration and shame. It makes me think a lot about Paul's letter in 2 Corinthians 12:9 in which he appeals to the Lord to help him overcome his struggles. God's reply always moves me: "My grace is sufficient for you, for power is made perfect in weakness."

What strikes me about the journey of Naman is his journey. He's believed to have had leprosy, a skin condition that many at that time thought meant a person was unclean or sinful or cursed. The king was likely concerned his leprosy would affect his ability to lead his army. And so, he sent him off to find a cure. To do something. I know when I got my diagnosis, I felt unclean, cursed . . . as though I was being punished. I too would have gone on a great journey to have God wave His arms and fix it. This was Naman's expectation as well.

But God's prophet, Elisha, rebukes Naman, who ultimately learns that God is not a magician, nor are His prophets. We are made whole through our faith, not magic. While it may be easy to conflate miracles and magic, they are not the same thing. Miracles are signs of God's faithfulness in our lives, and a testament to our own faith in Him.

The stories in the Bible call us to a life of faith. Not empty sacrifices, but *faith.* It reminds us that no matter the struggle or the trauma we are facing, there is more to this life than suffering. That joy and the peace that Elisha blesses Naman with come through faith and following God's guidance for our lives.

Two hundred and eighty miles may seem like a long distance to walk to find healing, but it is worth it, as Naman's

WHAT'S IN YOUR JOURNEY BACKPACK?

Item #9: I have been in a lot of different places in my wellness journey. Sometimes it's hard to figure out where exactly you might be struggling. Completing a Personal Wellness Assessment can help you identify where you struggle the most, and how to build goals in that area of your life.

story shows us. God makes us whole, body and soul, and this is only possible through faith. Yes, medicine has healed much of my body, but the way I have found wholeness is through my faith. Faith that God can use my broken body to do good. Faith that should I get sick again, God will care for my family. Faith that God is with me in every anxiety, fear, and uncertainty. That God is in all those parts that are still struggling.

We need to remember that our God is not a magician. God is a God of love, mercy, grace, and presence in the worst parts of our life and the Giver of wholeness when things will never be whole again. And all God wants in return is our faith and trust. So, go in peace. You are not alone.

THOUGHTS TO PONDER

1. Have you ever prayed that God would just wave a God wand and fix things?
2. Has there been benefits, growth, lessons through your struggles? Do you see God in those moments?
3. Do you find peace knowing that God is with you in those struggles or do you struggle to find God when things are hardest?

Steps taken: ____________ Miles journeyed: ____________

Exercise chosen: ____________________________________

Something I thought about:

____

____

____

____

Something I need to pray about:

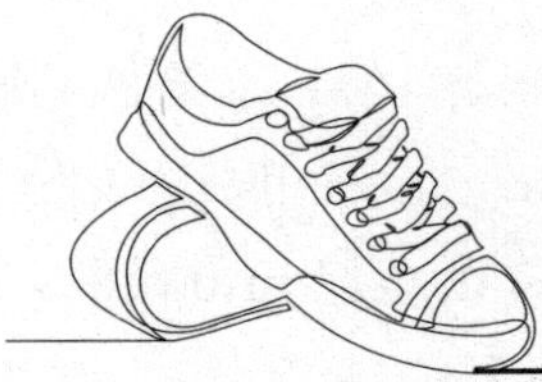

Day
10

A Return from Exile

In the first year of King Cyrus of Persia, in order that the word of the Lord by the mouth of Jeremiah might be accomplished, the Lord stirred up the spirit of King Cyrus of Persia so that he sent a herald throughout all his kingdom, and also in a written edict declared: "Thus says King Cyrus of Persia: The Lord, the God of heaven, has given me all the kingdoms of the earth, and he has charged me to build him a house at Jerusalem in Judah. Any of those among you who are of his people—may their God be with them!—are now permitted to go up to Jerusalem in Judah, and rebuild the house of the Lord, the God of Israel—he is the God who is in Jerusalem.

The heads of the families of Judah and Benjamin, and the priests and the Levites—everyone whose spirit God had stirred—got ready to go up and rebuild the house of the Lord in Jerusalem.

—Ezra 1:1–3, 5

BABYLON, PERSIA, TO JUDAH, ISRAEL: About 500 miles

The biblical commentary on this passage is fascinating.* Sometimes, reading the Bible, especially the Old Testament, through the lens of history, the cultural differences among the lands in which the stories take place, and the context of the political and religious conflicts of the times put God's story into a very different perspective. It also helps me to read commentary when I don't quite understand what a passage is trying to convey.

And yet, if we look at these stories, no matter how difficult they may be to understand, in the time, place, and geography in which they happened, we continue to see God. The closer we draw ourselves to God is where we find deeper understanding, deeper faith, and deeper appreciation for the breadth and depth of God over time and space. And it is in those moments when we realize that maybe we're a bit like the characters in the Bible—even kings, like Cyrus.

What stuck out to me when I first read the story of Cyrus was, "The Lord moved the heart of Cyrus." I've had my heart moved, but I don't think the moving of my heart is quite the same as God moving Cyrus's. I'm not a king. I don't live in a

---

* See Ellicott's Commentary for English Readers, MacLaren Expositions of Holy Scripture, and Matthew Henry's Concise Commentary at www.biblehub.com.

war-torn land. I am not a polytheist. I don't want to conquer anyone. I don't have a lot in common with Cyrus, but I do know what it's like to have my heart moved.

I remember specifically when I lost my hearing and was struggling with my disability. I was so alone. I used to play the piano. I used to sing. I used to listen to music. Now those things were gone. Even the comforting words of the liturgy I used to listen to every Sunday were lost to me. I was so angry. I remember the hot feeling in my cheeks, the tears that were streaming from my eyes, the rapid beating of my heart, and the feeling that I was coming out of my skin. It was intolerably uncomfortable (especially being in church where I was supposed to "behave"). But, in that moment, God showed up. I've never felt such love and comfort all of a sudden, out of the blue. No longer was I alone. And God said to me, "Anna,

WHAT'S IN YOUR JOURNEY BACKPACK?

Item #10: The Bible Hub app. Sometimes God's word is confusing to me. I am not sure what's being said in the context of the big picture. The Bible Hub app collates biblical commentary from leading scholars to help deepen my understanding of God's Word. Any other Bible apps of your preference should work and most allow you to listen to scripture through audio capabilities. So, throw your headphones on and listen to the Word of God as you do your daily walk.

you don't have to hear the Word of God. You have to *live* the Word of God." And since then, I've never been the same. My heart was moved.

To me, when the heart is moved, it is touched by compassion and understanding. It's illuminated by the knowledge that the world is greater than the small part of which I know. When the heart is stirred toward an awareness of God, awe takes over. And it is from that awe that we are able to have faith, that change occurs.

I think this story of Cyrus is a story of change. I don't think we see it all at once. But I think it demonstrates that God works through many people and places to move forward his plan for redemption of the world. God moves all sorts of hearts to make that happen. Today, God is moving your heart, because you too have a role in the redemption of the world.

THOUGHTS TO PONDER

1. Have you had your heart moved by God?
2. How did it impact you or your life?
3. Do you think you are a different person when you let God move your heart toward one of faith, hope, and love?

Steps taken: ____________ Miles journeyed: ____________

Exercise chosen: ____________________________________

Something I thought about:

____

____

____

____

Something I need to pray about:

____

____

____

____

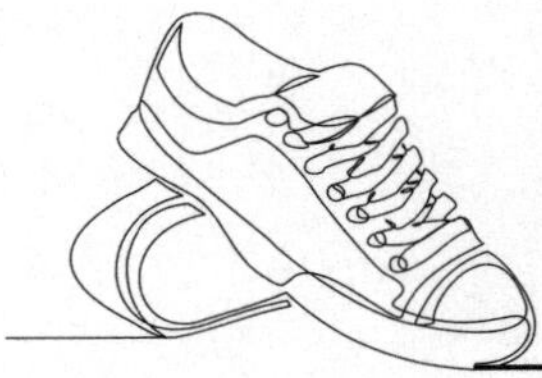

Part II

Exploring the New Testament

Day 11

The Magi Go East

In the time of King Herod, after Jesus was born in Bethlehem of Judea, wise men from the East came to Jerusalem, asking, "Where is the child who has been born king of the Jews? For we observed his star at its rising, and have come to pay him homage."

—Matthew 2:1–2

BABYLON (PRESUMED) TO JERUSALEM: 1,678 miles (about 3 to 4 months on foot/camel)

How far would you go to seek out the Messiah? What distance would you go? What struggle would you endure to get a glimpse of God? The Magi were presumably men from different nations and kingdoms who together sought out the infant Jesus. Some scholars believe they represent scholars from Persia, Arabia, and India who wanted to learn more about the Christ child. As the popular story goes, the three Magi, or "wise men," brought gifts of gold, frankincense, and myrrh to the Holy Family. Theologians have interpreted these gifts as symbolic: The gold signifies a king has come; frankincense, which was burned as incense in temples, points to the child's divinity; and lastly myrrh, which was used at the time to anoint the dead, foreshadows the great self-sacrifice that the baby, Jesus, would grow up to make for the sake of the world.

WHAT'S IN YOUR JOURNEY BACKPACK?

Item #11: Have you experienced trauma? If so, that can be an incredible burden and weight. The work of the Boulder Crest Foundation for Postraumatic Growth has been transformational for many individuals. I encourage you to seek out others that have experienced trauma and the process toward growth and healing.

This story reminds me of a major takeaway from the book of Psalms and Proverbs: "Wise men (and women) seek God." Like the Magi, you, too, are seeking Jesus, embarking on arduous spiritual and even physical journeys to draw closer to God. Your struggles are turned to strength when you seek God in the midst of ugly times, places, and people. Even as you tread unknown paths over great distances, rest assured that the destination will be worth it. The savior of the world awaits you.

After all, as we kick off our New Testament journeys, you will notice that they are all about the road to Jesus, redemption, healing, and being made whole. Our lives are all about the journey we take to care for ourselves, body and soul, and how we must push ourselves physically and spiritually toward the promises of Jesus.

I challenge you from this step forward, with every movement you make with your body, with every spiritual discipline you practice, to search for how your steps move you closer to God and to the awesome realization that you are marked as Jesus's own forever.

THOUGHTS TO PONDER

1. Is my journey in life reflective of one walking toward Christ or away?
2. What actions can I talk in my daily walk with God to bring me closer to God?
3. Are God's teachings and guidance for life things that I practice daily? Can those habits be improved?

Steps taken:___________ Miles journeyed:___________

Exercise chosen:_________________________________

Something I thought about:

____

____

____

____

Something I need to pray about:

____

____

____

____

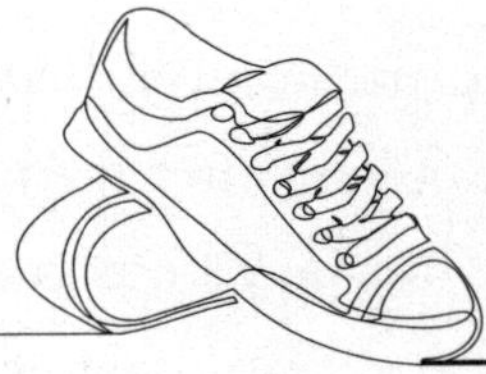

Day 12

The Flight into Egypt

Now after they had left, an angel of the Lord appeared to Joseph in a dream and said, "Get up, take the child and his mother, and flee to Egypt, and remain there until I tell you; for Herod is about to search for the child, to destroy him." Then Joseph got up, took the child and his mother by night, and went to Egypt, and remained there until the death of Herod. This was to fulfil what had been spoken by the Lord through the prophet, "Out of Egypt I have called my son."

—Matthew 2:13–15

NAZARETH TO EGYPT: Approximately 518 miles

In the Bible, the people of God were not strangers to dreams, and Joseph was no exception. Not long after the birth of Jesus, an angel of the Lord comes to Mary's husband in a dream and warns him that King Herod is seeking to murder Jesus. The angel then advises Joseph to take his family and seek refuge in Egypt.

This dream must have been scary for a number of reasons. First, Herod is planning to murder a child! In order to maintain his position as tetrarch, the king has convinced himself that he must commit infanticide. But this dream is also scary for another reason: Joseph and his young family are forced to flee to Egypt, a land in which the Jews were historically enslaved.

Sometimes, the warnings God send us may make us really uncomfortable or even fearful and may take us to scary places. But for me, these warnings demonstrate God's faithfulness. He wants to protect us, and in order for Him do so, we must trust in Him.

And so Joseph uproots his young and vulnerable family from Bethlehem and flees into Egypt. He trusts God's message, not doubting it for a second, and takes a leap of faith by venturing into a nation that had once been very cruel to his people. Why does he do this? Well, Joseph understands that even if the journey seems long, hard, and fraught with danger, He trusts that God has a greater plan for him and his family. A plan to protect them, to shield them from Herod's threats on their lives.

As I reflect on this story, I realize that God has turned my own path from one direction to another on multiple occasions to steer me away from danger. God has done—and is doing this—in your life as well, even if you have not noticed it. You always have the free will to choose, but many times the closing of doors is God's way of leading you back to Jesus and toward a better future for yourself.

I have no reason to believe that God is anything other than faithful and true to God's word. My experience, and the experience of thousands of believers before me, testify that if we search for God's will in our lives through prayer, study, discipline and discernment, we will become aware of the

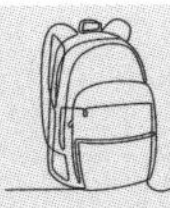

WHAT'S IN YOUR JOURNEY BACKPACK?

Item #12: Insight Timer app. My path to discernment is sometimes through prayer. Other times, it's through a meditative practice that allows me not to talk but to focus my intent on a specific idea or on God alone. The various practices available in Insight Timer provide guided tracks to explore a variety of different aspects of God and also of life. There are several other trusted meditation apps for you to choose from, so get meditating as you walk.

warnings and directions, so that we too can take action and make choices toward the paths that lead us to Jesus.

I like to think that Jesus comes to each and every one of us when we need it. "We do not know the hour or time of His coming," but when we study, when we pray, when we discern, we help ourselves prepare for that time.

THOUGHTS TO PONDER

1. Have you had warnings in your life that felt like they were from someone else? How did you respond to those warnings?
2. Looking back, do you think those warnings directed you in a better way than you could have decided for yourself?
3. Are you at a crossroads now searching for guidance? Look to prayer, study, and discernment for God's guidance at this point in your life.

Steps taken: ____________ Miles journeyed: ____________

Exercise chosen: ____

Something I thought about:

____

____

____

____

Something I need to pray about:

____

____

____

____

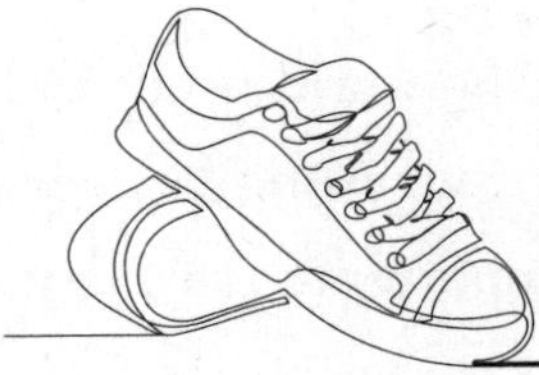

Day 13

The Traveling Preacher

He left Nazareth and made his home in Capernaum by the lake, in the territory of Zebulun and Naphtali, so that what had been spoken through the prophet Isaiah might be fulfilled:

"Land of Zebulun, land of
Naphtali,
on the road by the sea,
across the Jordan, Galilee of the
Gentiles—
the people who sat in darkness
have seen a great light,
and for those who sat in the
region and shadow of
death
light has dawned."

Matthew 4:13–16

NAZARETH TO CAPERNAUM: 30 miles

Everyone has a message that the world needs to hear. Whether it's for your family, your workplace, or even your nation, you have something important to say. Jesus certainly did, though His message—the message of salvation—was for the entire world.

You'll notice in this story that Jesus retreats or "withdraws" to Galilee. As Jesus shows us here, sometimes journeys aren't epic and exciting; sometimes they call us to introspection, meditation, and solitude.

For many of us, retreating someplace quiet allows us to shut out the noise of the world and hear God's word and guidance for that which we were called to do. While I don't have the flexibility to take off into the desert, or an abbey, to retreat and remove myself from the world, deepening my prayer practice and studying God's word has allowed me to find inner peace. Like you, I have a job, family, friends, obligations, but I cannot help but think that the practices that Jesus encourages, like prayer, study, and exercise, provide us with opportunities to focus our attention inwardly, to hear God. Sometimes going away doesn't simply indicate a miles-long journey. Rather, it refers to withdrawing into an internal place where you can hear God's voice more fully over the din of the world.

Like many people during the pandemic, I struggled with anger, depression, fear, and sorrow. Politics were divisive.

There was death, disease, despair, and uncertainty. In all of this, I wanted to lash out or curl up in a ball and shut out the world. I was just so tired. But soon I realized that this was not God's will for me. I had to rise to my feet and get moving—phyically and spiritually.

During that dark time, I had two things I could do within the confines of quarantine: walk and pray. Sometimes I would walk and not know what to pray, so I just walked. But this in itself was a spiritual activity, as I found that the fog in mind was beginning to lift. As I walked, I took on the habit of listening to scripture. And soon I found that the people of the Bible, too, had to deal with death, despair, illnesses, mean people, terrible politics, and angry mobs.

As I continued to listen to these histories, the Bible kept demonstrating the power of prayer and the importance of seeking God's will and not my own. I walked and walked

WHAT'S IN YOUR JOURNEY BACKPACK?

Item #13: *The Bible Recap* podcast. I love, love, love *The Bible Recap*. It explores one passage of the Bible for 365 days of the year, so it's perfect to have on hand for a daily walk. The Bible was originally an oral history, told by word of mouth, so it's powerful to listen to the words instead of simply reading them. What's better is that there are plenty of enriching podcasts on the Bible that you can listen to as you walk.

and prayed and prayed, beseeching God for His guidance, healing, good health, connectedness, kindness, and peace. I prayed to God to give me the strength to turn the other cheek, to love my neighbor, and to choose a different reaction than numbness, anger, and discord.

Through following God's guidance in my life, I found healing. While prayer didn't take away the trauma of the pandemic, the hurt, or what happened, choosing to go a different route and focus on God's word allowed me to find restoration.

Sometimes we need to go away to hear God's word. It doesn't mean you have to take a thirty-mile journey to a different location, but perhaps it means stepping back from that which you are struggling, to seek insight and guidance before reacting. Withdrawing often calls us to turn to God. And while our kneejerk reaction is to look for human solutions, prayer, exercise, and communing with God is often the only way we can truly find healing.

THOUGHTS TO PONDER

1. Do you have something that the world needs to hear? What is it?
2. Have you struggled between what God is trying to share with you vs. what the world wants you to think?
3. What are some things you can do to better hear God's Word and your voice?

Steps taken: ____________ Miles journeyed: ____________

Exercise chosen: ____________________________________

Something I thought about:

____

____

____

____

Something I need to pray about:

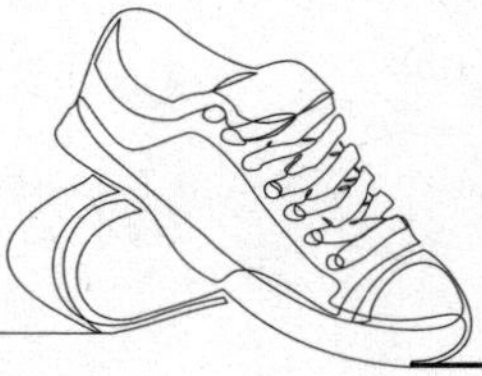

Day 14

On the Mountain with Jesus

When Jesus saw the crowds, he went up the mountain; and after he sat down, his disciples came to him. Then he began to speak, and taught them, saying:

"Blessed are the poor in spirit, for theirs is the kingdom of heaven.

"Blessed are those who mourn, for they will be comforted.

"Blessed are the meek, for they will inherit the earth.

"Blessed are those who hunger and thirst for righteousness, for they will be filled.

"Blessed are the merciful, for they will receive mercy.

"Blessed are the pure in heart, for they will see God.

"Blessed are the peacemakers, for they will be called children of God.

"Blessed are those who are persecuted for righteousness' sake, for theirs is the kingdom of heaven.

"Blessed are you when people revile you and persecute you and utter all kinds of evil against you falsely on my account. Rejoice and be glad, for your reward is great in heaven, for in the same way they persecuted the prophets who were before you."

—Matthew 5:1–12

GALILEE TO CAPERNAUM: 25-ish miles

In the public health literature on writing health policy, publishing standards and implementing evidenced-based practice are essential to making positive change in population health outcomes. Evidence suggests on small scale (individual) and large scale (population) levels that when we write down goals, objectives, and a plan, we are more likely to be successful in achieving the goals we set.

We don't ever seem to do this practice in our personal, spiritual, or faith lives. It's rare that individuals think about the kind of Christian they want to be and set goals for working toward the life they want to lead in their faith journey. And I think we do a disservice to ourselves when we don't think about the standards we want to uphold in specific situations, when we don't think about how we want to face the worst days in our lives, and when we don't practice skills and

WHAT'S IN YOUR JOURNEY BACKPACK?

Item #14: If you have nutrition-based wellness goals, my go-to app is MyFitnessPal. It will help you identify fuel-based needs, macros, and eating plans based on your lifestyle. Find a fitness app that works for you and get started today! It's never too late to get healthy.

disciplines that help us to live these Christian standards on a day-to-day basis.

We often believe that because we have faith that Christian standards will just come to us. But belief does not alone generate habit. I believe that a diet of donuts and pizza is bad for me, but if I do not *practice* moderation, self-control, and discipline, then my flawed self will reach for what is easy and yummy. I will then regret how I did not make a choice that aligned with my belief.

Our faith is similar. Daily prayer, meditation, scripture reading, and writing out the practices that can help lead us closer to God are essential to successfully integrating these habits into practice. After all, while your faith and God's love are *always* there, especially in your darkest hour, it is easy to feel as though God has abandoned and left you if you do not flex your spiritual muscles. Cultivating God's grace takes practice, and it means practicing those tenets of faith in the day-to-day. To me, the Beatitudes help us identify areas of our spiritual lives where we need to focus in order to lead holy lives. Jesus calls us to follow Him on His journey up to the Mount and to be merciful, to be peacemakers, to be meek, and to pursue righteousness. Those are spiritual practices that take work.

I never understood people who said their faith was easy. I guess my belief in God came easy, but my faith is a whole different animal. It takes work because, if I'm being honest,

I'm lazy at heart. I don't want to practice. I don't want to turn the other cheek. I want to choose the easy way of donuts and pizza, my identity, my way, my likes, my desires. But my way is not God's way, so I need to work. To get disciplined. And in the end I know it will all be worth it.

THOUGHTS TO PONDER

1. What would be your natural inclination in your life if you didn't practice the standards of Christian living? Be honest!
2. What are habits you think you need to practice to focus your self more fully on God?
3. Are there things you have done in the moment of being faced with evil, loss, degradation, anger that you wish you could have responded differently?
4. What is your hope for the future in your Christian life?

Steps taken:__________ Miles journeyed:__________

Exercise chosen:____________________

Something I thought about:

____

____

____

____

Something I need to pray about:

____

____

____

____

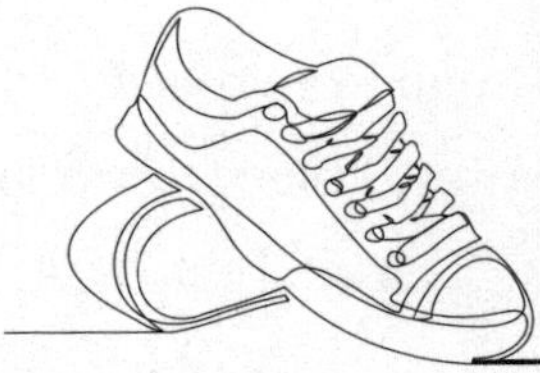

Day 15

Stepping into the Healing Pools

Now in Jerusalem by the Sheep Gate there is a pool, called in Hebrew Beth-zatha, which has five porticoes. In these lay many invalids—blind, lame, and paralysed. One man was there who had been ill for thirty-eight years. When Jesus saw him lying there and knew that he had been there a long time, he said to him, "Do you want to be made well?" The sick man answered him, "Sir, I have no one to put me into the pool when the water is stirred up; and while I am making my way, someone else steps down ahead of me." Jesus said to him, "Stand up, take your mat and walk." At once the man was made well, and he took up his mat and began to walk.

—John 5:1–9

THE JOURNEY TO THE HEALING POOL: Unknown. Approximately 10–20 feet

In my mind's eye, I can see the sick man from this story lying by the pool. The waters are clear and blue, shimmering under the hot sun. There are stony steps leading up to it. The pool is right there, just a bit beyond the man's reach. There are people bustling around, passing him by, busy on their own journeys. But this man cannot walk. And so he is ignored. Perhaps unseen. How often do you think, when you are not doing well spiritually or physically, that you are invisible? As I envision the man lying near the pool, I think he is maybe ten to twenty steps away. He is close, yet so far.

History tells us that a number of things are happening in this scene. First, Jewish tradition engaged in bathing as a symbolic means of healing and cleansing the body for sanctification. Second, cultural traditions held that certain baths and pools were sacred for their healing properties. It was believed that certain waters held spiritual properties that aided in the healing of afflictions. Third, people did not stop and help the sick because they were afraid that by doing so that they, too, would become "unclean." They believed that touching the ill would tarnish them. After all, at the time, disease was considered an outward manifestation of inward spiritual disease and sin.

While we know more now, there are several things that society has in common today with that of our ancestors. Illness and disease still have a certain amount of stigma. People often wonder what someone "did wrong" to get their illnesses. In fact, we ourselves often think that if we had "done something right," then we would not have gotten sick. It is a poisonous mindset, and one that offers no relief and healing. We are also guilty of looking the other way when the poor and the sick are at our feet. We walk by without stopping to help them into the proverbial pool. The sick, unfortunately, are still invisible.

But Jesus sees the sick. As soon as He spots the man suffering near the pool, He orders him to get up and walk. In my opinion, there are many layers to this command. On the surface, Jesus is literally telling the man to stand on his two feet, to get moving. On a deeper level, Jesus is insisting that the man take control of his destiny, to not only step into the pool without relying on another's assistance but to start his own journey of healing.

When I was younger, this parable—and other parables about healing—troubled me greatly. I used to feel that I did not

WHAT'S IN YOUR JOURNEY BACKPACK?

Item #15 Music! When I'm not listening to scripture or a podcast on my walk, I'm listening to some song that makes me want to jump and dance! If you've never listened to Fernando Ortega's acoustic rendition of "Praise to the Lord, the Almighty," you are missing out. Music makes walking so much more bearable and even fun.

have enough faith because my illness and disability remained. Praying, "getting up and walking," and loving God never changed my physical reality. I often felt that I must have had something wrong with me or my faith because there wasn't a magic wand of faith that just "fixed it."

When I reflect back on this journey of the sick man to the healing pools, my perception of what Jesus is teaching is now different. Jesus does not only heal people; He also tells them to *do* something. For instance, He tells the sick man to "get up." This order is one of action. It is an order to make a choice and *go.* It's an order to be active in your healing process and not just sit back and let things happen.

In your own life, in your own journey, there is a decision point. No matter what route you choose, you first have to get up and take that first step. That step is your decision to address the goals you have made for yourself and the troubles with which you are wrestling. The journey to the healing pool in this story was not a long one. But you cannot take a few steps in any direction without taking that first step. This is what we are doing today with the journey to the healing pool. With your prayer walk, listen to what Jesus is saying to you. Listen to your prayers and hear where your journey needs to take you. Then, *go.* Get up, take action, and keep putting one foot in front of the other.

THOUGHTS TO PONDER

1. Is there something in your life that you feel is right there but just out of reach? What is it?
2. Where do you hear Jesus calling you to take your personal mind, body, and spiritual journey in the next forty days?
3. What do you worry about on this journey?

Steps taken: ___________ Miles journeyed: ___________

Exercise chosen: ________________________________

Something I thought about:

____

____

____

____

Something I need to pray about:

____

____

____

____

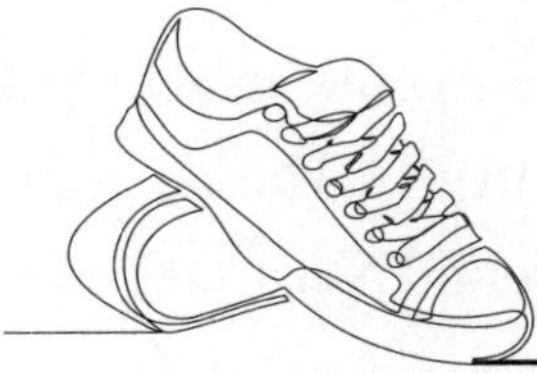

Day 16

Crossing the Stormy Sea

Immediately he made his disciples get into the boat and go on ahead to the other side, to Bethsaida, while he dismissed the crowd. After saying farewell to them, he went up on the mountain to pray. When evening came, the boat was out on the lake, and he was alone on the land. When he saw that they were straining at the oars against an adverse wind, he came towards them early in the morning, walking on the lake. He intended to pass them by. But when they saw him walking on the lake, they thought it was a ghost and cried out; for they all saw him and were terrified. But immediately he spoke to them and said, "Take heart, it is I; do not be afraid." Then he got into the boat with them and the wind ceased. And they were utterly astounded.

—Mark 6:45–52

NAZARETH TO BETHSAIDA: 32 miles

Warning: I am going to make some armchair theology assumptions in this entry. In Mark 6, Jesus and His disciples are hanging in and around Nazareth, no doubt stirring up trouble—good trouble—because that's my man Jesus for you. We know that He and the crew are heading from Nazareth to Bethsaida. By foot this journey is roughly thirty-two miles. However, if they cross the Sea of Kinnereth/ Sea of Galilee at Tiberius, they would save themselves some distance (maybe five to ten miles by foot) while letting the boat do some of the work for them. For whatever reason (okay, because Jesus told them to), the disciples leave Jesus on the shore while getting into the boat. Meanwhile, Jesus sits and watches as their boat sets off into the waters.

Anyway, the disciples are rowing when suddenly a storm hits them. We are told that they are fighting the wind, likely

WHAT'S IN YOUR JOURNEY BACKPACK?

Item #16: Coffee. While all things are possible for God, for me, very little is possible without coffee. It's definitely in my journey pack and gives me a boost when I need it. It's not a bad thing to enjoy the fruit of God's green earth, and boy am I glad He made coffee beans!

scared out of their wits, when Jesus comes to meet them. This makes me remember when I was a kid and my grandmother would holler at me to get out of the lake at the first sound of thunder or sight of lightning. But instead of hollering at the disciples to get out of the water, Jesus decides to start teaching.

Before we go into this teaching, I'd like to note something. If the disciples are in the middle of the lake, and the lake is presumably about ten miles wide, then Jesus walked on water for about five miles. My calves hurt at the thought. Have you ever walked on an uneven surface for any length of time? It's hard, and it hurts.

But this is Jesus we are talking about. Jesus goes. He walks. He does the unthinkable. This whole thing is so improbable that the disciples think He's a ghost, that He is unreal. Mark includes this in his narrative because the disciples have yet to comprehend the story of the loaves and fishes . . . they fail to understand what Jesus meant when He said, "Through God, all things are possible."

When I read this passage, I hear Jesus telling us to take that first step toward the impossible. Sometimes we need to believe that while we might not be able to make the impossible happen, through God, all things are possible. Even amid the storms of life, we can find shelter and safety and hope. So, when you are going through it, look into the distance. Look past the fog and the rain and see. Jesus is approaching you, traversing the waves, His arms outstretched, ready to catch you.

THOUGHTS TO PONDER

1. Are you baffled by God's work in your life right now?
2. What do you think this story is teaching you about the changes you are trying to make in your life?
3. What do you think of the idea that "through God, all things are possible?"

Steps taken:__________ Miles journeyed:__________

Exercise chosen:____________________

Something I thought about:

____

____

____

____

Something I need to pray about:

____

____

____

____

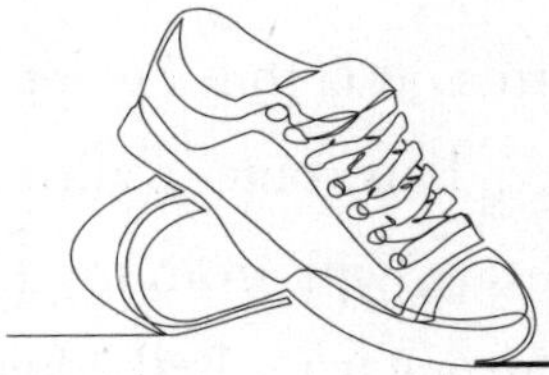

Day 17

The Journey from Bethlehem to Jerusalem

Jesus went throughout Galilee, teaching in their synagogues and proclaiming the good news of the kingdom and curing every disease and every sickness among the people. So his fame spread throughout all Syria, and they brought to him all the sick, those who were afflicted with various diseases and pains, demoniacs, epileptics, and paralytics, and he cured them. And great crowds followed him from Galilee, the Decapolis, Jerusalem, Judea, and from beyond the Jordan.

—Matthew 4:23–25

BETHLEHEM TO JERUSALEM: 90 miles

I knew when I sat down to write this book that I wanted to speak about the Bethlehem route. This route inspired the Bethlehem challenge, a five-mile-a-day walk from my *Christ Walk* series that represents Jesus's journey from Bethlehem to Jerusalem—from birth to death.

Anyway, as I often do, I usually head out to do some sort of exercise when I need to muddle through my thoughts. The majority of my brilliant ideas come when my body is in motion, and one particular day was no different. I had been trying out spinning. I was not very good at it, and I did not have a fancy bike, but I'd hop on it two to three times a week for a spin. On that day, the instructor was just amazeballs. Her spirit and joy

WHAT'S IN YOUR JOURNEY BACKPACK?

Item #17: The Peloton app. If you didn't guess from the dialogue with the spin instructor, I am an avid fan of the Peloton app. I don't have a fancy bike, but I will use the app for a bicycle workout. The instructors are enthusiastic, it's hard to be in a bad mood afterward, and it's an incredible cardiovascular exercise routine. There are so many online fitness companions, so I encourage you to try one out. I promise you will feel refreshed and invigorated after using it.

and encouragement had me shouting out enthusiastically during the ride. When she'd call for me to up the resistance on the bike, I would shout in a loud voice, "I've got this baby. No one is taking me down!" I sang. I grunted. I hollered. I shouted. I cried a little, too. At one point, the instructor said something really profound: "How hard will you challenge yourself to be transformed? How hard will you work to be changed?"

This was my lightbulb moment. Jesus was working *hard* throughout His thirty-something years. He was working and challenging Himself and reaching out to people in need. He was touching the sick, the blind, the lame, the dirty, the traitorous, the poor. He was walking from Galilee, to Jerusalem, to Bethsaida, to Nazareth, Capernaum, and all around. He was blazing a path to make a difference and change the world forever.

How hard will you challenge yourself to be changed? How hard will you work to make a difference in the world? Where will you go on your journey that will make you push yourself just a little harder and a little farther? Whenever I talk to people about choosing physical, spiritual, mental goals, I always ask them to choose something a little outside of their comfort zone and be creative in how they will get to where they want to go. Just like Jesus was transformed as He journeyed from Bethlehem to Jerusalem, you'll be transformed when you accept a challenge and rise up to meet it.

Don't be afraid to push yourself outside of your comfort zone. I am fairly sure that Jesus was outside of His comfort zone from time to time. Can you imagine being a twelve-year-old child walking into the Temple, sitting down with the elders and essentially conducting a midrash with them (Luke 2:41–52)? This is equivalent to a preteen walking into a graduate-level university class and holding their own. That is pretty impressive. We also know that education transforms people, so as Jesus is learning, He is absorbing and being transformed by the teachings of His elders.

When we go to Jerusalem with Jesus, we encounter the cross, which is literally two physical lines that intersect each other. The point at which these two things meet is transformational. You cannot have the promise of the resurrection without the potential of something more. And that potential for something more is the promise from God that there *is more.* Suffering is not the end of the story; transformation is.

You may be going through a period of physical, spiritual, and/or mental suffering on your walk. One of the messages of Jesus's journey from Bethlehem to Jerusalem is that if you work through the suffering to seek purpose and meaning, then you too will be a transformed individual.

THOUGHTS TO PONDER

1. Are you currently undergoing challenges in your life?
2. How are you rising up to meet those challenges?
3. What are ways you can step out of your comfort zone?

Steps taken: ____________ Miles journeyed: ____________

Exercise chosen: ____________________________________

Something I thought about:

____

____

____

____

Something I need to pray about:

____

____

____

____

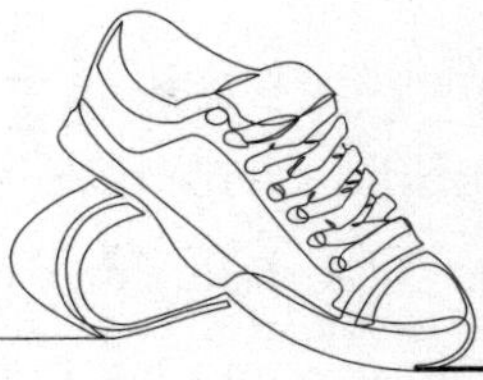

Day

18

The Disciples Venture Out

He called the twelve and began to send them out two by two, and gave them authority over the unclean spirits. He ordered them to take nothing for their journey except a staff; no bread, no bag, no money in their belts; but to wear sandals and not to put on two tunics. He said to them, "Wherever you enter a house, stay there until you leave the place. If any place will not welcome you and they refuse to hear you, as you leave, shake off the dust that is on your feet as a testimony against them." So they went out and proclaimed that all should repent. They cast out many demons, and anointed with oil many who were sick and cured them.

—Mark 6:7–13

NAZARETH TO CANA: 5–6 miles
NAZARETH TO NAIN: 10 miles
NAZARETH TO TIBERIAS: 18 miles
NAZARETH TO MAGDALA: 23 miles

In Mark 1–6, Jesus and the disciples are teaching in Jesus's hometown of Nazareth. Some of the surrounding towns include Cana, Nain, Tiberias, and Magdala. To give you some context of distance, Cana is approximately five miles from Nazareth, and Tiberius is roughly eighteen miles away. So, the disciples are traveling—mostly on foot!—anywhere from five to ten miles a day. Those are a lot of miles!

As I try to imagine myself in these journeys, I notice a number of things. First off, it's hot. The roads are dusty. There is no Sirius XM blasting on the radio to make the journey easier. There is just you . . . and your companion. What strikes me most about this story is that Jesus didn't send the disciples

WHAT'S IN YOUR JOURNEY BACKPACK?

Item #18: Make a friend! Okay, okay, so you can't quite put a friend in a backpack, I know. But whether I'm using Strava, Fitbit, MapMyRun, or any other fitness app, there's a place where you can find a companion to join you on your walk. There's nothing quite like having your journey cheered on by a friend as you record your miles, so I urge you to find someone. Having a partner on your walk or run would certainly make it more enjoyable.

out alone. He sent them in pairs. This tells me *so* much about Jesus and people. Jesus knows we need each other. In fact, sociological evidence suggests that when people are making change, they are more successful when they have a partner or a group to support them in their efforts. Jesus knows we are a communal species, that we belong together. He sends us out with a companion because He doesn't want us to feel alone. After all, a miles-long journey can be hard and lonely. Jesus knows we need people.

You need people too. Whether you are an introvert or an extrovert, you are called to live in community. We experience the trials of others in community, and this helps us develop love and compassion. When we share our own experiences, we let other people know that they are not alone in their journey. When we live in community, we reach out to others so that they too can be enfolded into a circle of love as well. Living in circles of community that focus on love, compassion, and support creates ripple effects. Each pair of disciples that Jesus sent out to spread the Good News was just like a rock skipping in a pond. Every rock created ripple effects that helped countless others make necessary and pivotal changes in their communities and their world.

As you go on this forty-day journey, think of someone to bring along the way. They don't have to be physically present on the walk with you, but let them in on the changes or goals you have set for yourself. Your invitation may call them to focus on things they need to change in their lives. So, go ahead! Be the ripple that creates a shockwave of change in their life. Jesus isn't sending you out on this journey alone; He's asking you to invite others to join you, to come along as you make a difference in the world.

THOUGHTS TO PONDER

1. Who could you invite on this journey?
2. What would you like to tell them about your journey?
3. Are there things you'd like for them to help you with on this journey?

Steps taken: __________ Miles journeyed: __________

Exercise chosen: ______________________________

Something I thought about:

____

____

____

____

Something I need to pray about:

____

____

____

____

Day

19

Resting at the Well

But he had to go through Samaria. So he came to a Samaritan city called Sychar, near the plot of ground that Jacob had given to his son Joseph. Jacob's well was there, and Jesus, tired out by his journey, was sitting by the well. It was about noon.

—John 4:4–6

GALILEE TO SYCHAR, SAMARIA: Approximately 36 miles

"Jesus was tired." This section of the passage about Jesus and the Samaritan woman discussing the water of life is awe-striking to me. Jesus was *tired.* I resonate deeply with His vulnerable display of humanness. I too get tired. Frequently. I am easily worn out in my day-to-day life, and so I pray and meditate on hope. I do not want to be consumed by the epidemic of hopelessness that seems to be coming from media, politics, contention, and strife. These four things are the new Horsemen of the Apocalypse. They tear down people, faith, and communities and sow discord, discontent, and disillusionment.

If you examine the period in which Jesus was preaching, He was dealing with all the same things. Sure, He didn't have a twenty-four-hour news service, but the town crier and gossip mill likely ran strong. The political environment was contentious between the haves and the have-nots. Whether it involved culture, politics, the military, and religion, contentions ran rampant. And, of course, there was strife. People were struggling with famine, judicial inequality, racism, culturalism, and so much more.

And yet, Jesus continued to preach forgiveness, compassion, and connection. As fully God, Jesus understood the big picture that the issues facing humanity were universal and could best be overcome by mutual understanding, respect, and love. But, as fully human, Jesus was tired.

I appreciate the human side of Jesus greatly. It makes our God approachable, real, personal. It makes me feel as though God really understands how difficult it is to be human. Jesus's humanness also gives me hope that it won't always be this way. There will come a better day. And God's consistency over time and generations assures me that although suffering is of the now, it isn't of the *always*.

Although Jesus was tired, He got up again. He continued to preach. He ministered to the Samaritan woman, sharing with her the message of eternal salvation, of the "living water" that permanently sates our thirst and refreshes our soul. His example ultimately teaches us that it is a good thing to pause,

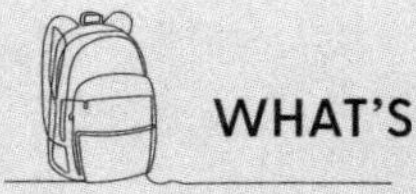

WHAT'S IN YOUR JOURNEY BACKPACK?

Item #19: Sleep. Sleep, activity, and nutrition are the three building blocks for strong cardiovascular health. And yet most Americans do not get enough sleep. If you are tired, getting decent sleep (7–8 hours/night) can help. Sleep heals. Our bodies do our work of repair at night, and if you aren't sleeping enough, you aren't giving your body time to heal mind, body, or spirit. The Abide app offers soothing meditations that can help lull you to bed, as well as invigorating meditations as you start your daily walk.

to take a break, to drink a cup of wine, to pray, to worship, and be refreshed with God's word. When we do this, we too can go back out in the world and share the love that God asks of us.

Ultimately, it's okay to be tired. In fact, when you are tired, that's a good sign. It means you can take a moment to rejuvenate yourself, to be intentional with caring for your body and soul. Make time for rest because God will inevitably call you out again. Our work here on earth is not done.

THOUGHTS TO PONDER

1. Do you struggle with being tired?
2. What makes you tired?
3. What do you think could refresh your soul?
4. How can you practice that a little bit at a time each day? Or each week?

Steps taken: ____________ Miles journeyed: ___________

Exercise chosen: ____________________________________

Something I thought about:

____

____

____

____

Something I need to pray about:

____

____

____

____

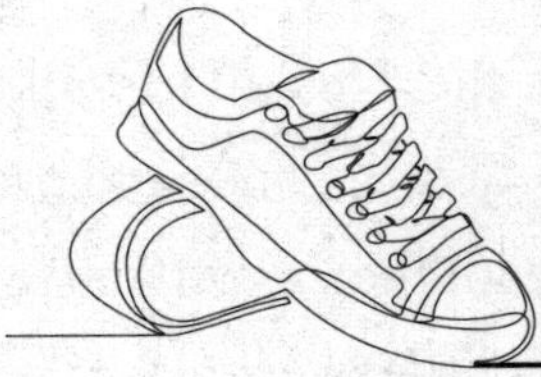

Day 20

The Way of the Cross

As they went out, they came upon a man from Cyrene named Simon; they compelled this man to carry his cross.

—Matthew 27:32

THE VIA DELAROSA **("THE WAY OF SUFFERING"):**
Roughly 2.2 miles

When Jesus was sentenced to die, He had to walk—or rather trek—to the cross. I sat down once and tried to map out a route that was consistent with the Passion narratives and came up with a route that was a little over two miles. It's not a terribly long distance. I've walked two miles at a time many, many times before. However, I wasn't walking with a broken body, a body that had been whipped and punched and beaten with closed fists. I didn't have on rags that chafed my skin. And I sure as heck wasn't barefoot or had on a crown made of prickly thorns drawing blood from my temples. I certainly didn't have a heavy cross to bear on my back.

When I think about the path Jesus walked to His crucifixion, aptly known as the *Via Dolorosa*—"the Way of Suffering"—I

WHAT'S IN YOUR JOURNEY BACKPACK?

Item #20: Daily gratitude. The brain is neuroplastic. If we feed it a steady diet of gratitude, we begin to look at the world through a lens that is positive, humble, and life-affirming. So, I encourage you to keep a daily gratitude journal. Whether it's in a book or a journal app, jot down what your thankful for every day before you walk and watch as your journeys become more peaceful.

always feel filled with gratitude. I think about my struggles and realize that many things could be much, much worse. But I also feel uncomfortable. It makes me realize that sometimes suffering is necessary if we wish to be transformed. To me, the cross represents the point at which suffering and transformation intersect. *Literally.* Without the cross, there is no transformation or suffering.

Those two miles were so difficult for Jesus to traverse that a man, Simon of Cyrene, was chosen by the Romans to help Jesus carry His cross. From what we can understand, Simon was a reluctant traveler on this journey. He didn't volunteer to help Jesus carry the cross but was chosen against his will. Can you imagine what was going through his mind? *Must I really help this convicted criminal, bloodied and smelly, bear his punishment?*

While the Bible does not refer to Simon's life following the crucifixion, tradition holds that he helped spread Christianity to Egypt and that Cyrenians were some of the first Christian believers. In fact, Mark 15:21 mentions that Simon's sons—Rufus and Alexander—were early Christians. Clearly, Simon's experience bearing Jesus's cross was positively life-changing.

Suffering can transform people in both bad and good ways, but Jesus reminds us that we have the ability to choose to follow God in that suffering. And in that choice is freedom. God has given us an amazing gift of love and because of that love we can be freed from the spiritual shackles that are weighing us down.

Walk 2.2 miles today. Meditate on suffering and love. Imagine Jesus next to you as you bear your proverbial cross. Imagine being called to walk in love and watch as your own suffering is transformed. Do that for forty days, and you will be changed. The Way of Suffering is also the Way of Love.

THOUGHTS TO PONDER

1. Have you ever needed help on a journey? Who came to your aid?
2. Take a moment to consider how suffering has transformed your life. What difficult experience did you undergo that made you a stronger, more godly person?
3. How can you be the "Simon of Cyrene" on another person's journey?

Steps taken: ____________ Miles journeyed: ____________

Exercise chosen: ____________________________________

Something I thought about:

____

____

____

____

Something I need to pray about:

Part III

Traveling with the Apostles

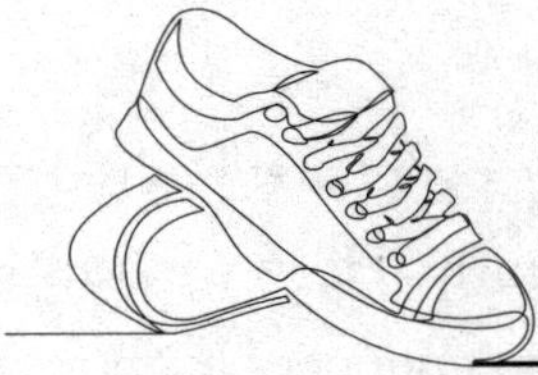

Day 21

The Road to Damascus

Meanwhile Saul, still breathing threats and murder against the disciples of the Lord, went to the high priest and asked him for letters to the synagogues at Damascus, so that if he found any who belonged to the Way, men or women, he might bring them bound to Jerusalem. Now as he was going along and approaching Damascus, suddenly a light from heaven flashed around him. He fell to the ground and heard a voice saying to him, "Saul, Saul, why do you persecute me?" He asked, "Who are you, Lord?" The reply came, "I am Jesus, whom you are persecuting. But get up and enter the city, and you will be told what you are to do." The men who were travelling with him stood speechless because they heard the voice but saw no one. Saul got up from the ground, and though his eyes were open, he could see nothing; so they led him by the hand and brought him into Damascus.

—Acts 9:1–8

JERUSALEM TO DAMASCUS: 203 miles

Jerusalem to Damascus is a little over two hundred miles. It is not a journey to take lightly. Here we find Paul, formerly Saul, who is seeking to persecute people of the Way. Men, women, children, families, and churches—he is rounding them all up and torturing them for their beliefs. If you think you've been terrorized for your beliefs, I do not think you really know what that means, particularly if you're living in modern America or Western Europe. Here, we lead pretty awesome lives because of our right to religious freedom. We should never, ever take that for granted.

Regardless of the brief political rabbit hole I fell into just now, what strikes me about this passage and journey is Jesus. Jesus is not afraid to say it like it is. Jesus is not afraid of what people think or being politically correct. He is not afraid of hurting peoples' feelings. "Hey, you, yes, you . . . you are a murderous thug!" Jesus is not just calling out Saul in this passage; He is calling out each and every one of us on our behaviors, whether big or small. This is another great reason why we need to study our Bible regularly. There are *so* many lessons in it that teach us how we can change our behavior and hear God's call in our own lives. You might not be a murderous thug, but Jesus is calling out to you. "Hey you!

Yes *you!* You need to change." Every one of us has something to work on in life.

Have you ever felt like Jesus was calling you and your behavior out? I have. I have heard Him tell me that I'm being selfish, greedy, gluttonous, uncharitable, mean, impatient, irreverent, and more. I have been rebuked in my prayers and while reading my Bible. I have felt in my body when I am veering away from a life that is in line with my Christian beliefs. God has made me aware of consistent, repetitious, and ongoing behaviors that are eating away at my soul and that are not in line with my Christian beliefs.

In fact, things that eat away at your soul often eat away at your physical body too. After all, when our soul or mind is

WHAT'S IN YOUR JOURNEY BACKPACK?

Item #21: Prayer (duh). If prayer isn't in your journey pack, what are you doing? Prayer and meditation are great practices to reduce stress. Stress contributes to inflammatory processes, which contribute to disease and illness. Things you can do to calm your nervous system are good things for your body. So, pray! Hallow is an excellent prayer and meditation app, though there are many others to pick from, if you prefer. If you have no words to pray—don't worry. Just plug your earphones in and listen to the prayers on a trusted app.

suffering, stress can and will invade our body. Stress creates a chemical reaction that releases all sorts of hormones that poison us. Depending on the person, stress can result in weight gain, increased blood pressure, increased blood sugar, higher resting heart rates, increased muscle tension, nerve compression, blurred vision, headaches, numbness, tingling, and a host of other symptoms that, if left untreated for long periods of time, can increase your risk for chronic health conditions, such as heart disease, lung disease, nerve disease, depression/anxiety, and many others. Some scientists posit that the rate of chronic illness we see in America today has a lot to do with our lifestyles and the choices we make with our bodies. Stress is a key factor.

Now, back to Damascus Road, where Saul is pretty stressed out himself. As the story goes, the man, having previously gone out on a rampage arresting Christians, has been struck blind. Now y'all know I know what it's like to lose a sense. It's terrifying! Imagine, one moment you can see and then—boom! You're blind. For three days Saul did not see. Each step he took had to be guided by another, and the only voice he heard was that of God. How the mighty had fallen!

Then God called Ananias, one of the people who Saul had persecuted, to heal Saul. I find it interesting that God worked not only in Saul's life, but also in the life of the persecuted one, Ananias, to create healing. God did not only heal God's people. God seeks healing in all people.

Now, ask yourself. Are you on the Damascus Road? Where is Jesus calling out to you? Will you let go and let God's grace and mercy transform you as Paul did? If so, what do you see at the end of the Damascus journey? Are you willing to overcome obstacles to become the person God meant you to be?

THOUGHTS TO PONDER

1. Are you on the Damascus Road?
2. What do you want to do on this journey?
3. Can you walk 203 miles to think about it during this time?
4. What would you like to see at the end of the Damascus Road?

Steps taken: ___________ Miles journeyed: ___________

Exercise chosen: ___________________________________

Something I thought about:

____

____

____

____

Something I need to pray about:

____

____

____

____

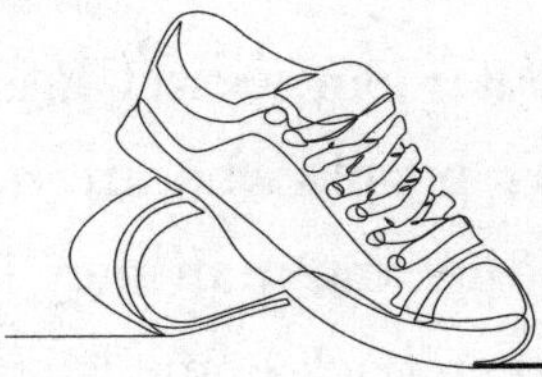

Day 22

Heading Back to Emmaus

Now on that same day two of them were going to a village called Emmaus, about seven miles from Jerusalem.

While they were talking and discussing, Jesus himself came near and went with them.

And he said to them, "What are you discussing with each other while you walk along?"

—Luke 24:13, 15, 17

EMMAUS TO JERUSALEM: 7 miles or 27 miles

The Road to Emmaus is a popular journey in Christian literature. It tells of ordinary people who are transformed forever when they realize that the man they have been interacting with on their journey back home is in fact the risen Jesus.

There are a couple of things about this journey that jump out at me. As someone who spends her time pouring over distances in the Bible to challenge myself and others to walk, run, swim, or bike their way through the Bible, this story intrigues me because it tells me that Emmaus to Jerusalem is seven miles.

Except . . .

When I search on Google Maps the distance, I am told that the route from Emmaus to Jersualem is closer to twenty-seven miles. Hmm. I get stuck in a quandary here. Do I recommend focusing on seven miles or twenty-seven miles? What is the writer trying to tell me about seven miles? We know that seven is a holy number in the Bible. We also know that it is highly unlikely that the original writers used mileage (a purely American atrocity of measure) when describing how far things were from one another. We know that what Google Maps calls Emmaus may not be the Emmaus of biblical times and that the number seven often indicated an ambiguous but large amount when describing time, place, people, and distances. If you have any sort of OCD, this sort of ambiguity probably drives you a little crazy.

However, what I would like for you to think about is not the correct distance but the journey itself. Whether seven miles or twenty-seven miles is the right thing for you, what matters is that you make the journey. Record where you will go, how far you will travel, how long it will take you to do it, and then do it! Note how you feel when you accomplish each mile, what you learned along the way. Remember: journeys are not necessarily about how long you travel or how far you go but the transformation and change that occur along the way.

Now, back to the journey. The disciples are walking miles to Jerusalem. Jesus is dead. They are alone. The passage mentions they were sad, their faces sullen. Imagine how disheartened they must have felt. The One they believed to be the Messiah was dead—executed brutally by the Romans. They are so distraught, in fact, that they leave Jerusalem and go back to Emmaus, presumably their hometown. It's a "backward" journey, if I may, a return home after a painful defeat. The disciples no longer see any point in staying in Jerusalem, where the Messiah was destined to triumphantly come. I wonder how many "backward" journeys we are tempted to go on when we feel like our journey is no longer worth it.

Now, imagine this.

When the disciples realize that the mysterious man they've invited to dinner is Jesus—the risen Jesus—they are so stunned that they *return* to Jerusalem and proclaim to the other disciples that Jesus is alive, is risen! What a story! Imagine—they had given up. Their Messiah was gone. Reality wasn't playing out how they had envisioned. Their journey wasn't going the way they wanted.

But the passage goes on to say, "While they were discussing these things, Jesus Himself arrived and joined them on their journey." Holy Reeboks, my friends! Have you ever been walking along, chatting to yourself or to a companion, feeling all the feels, and all of a sudden it just felt like Jesus is right there, right then? I know I have. Obviously, it is a spiritual feeling, but sometimes there is a whisper in my head during these walks, a whisper that makes me realize that God is present with me always, guiding and loving me and giving me peace.

I am deeply thankful that God joins us on our journeys. I find that I often have to still my mind or let it run loose at the beginning of my walk, enter active prayer as I sort through the muddle of emotions and thoughts at the middle, and be silent so I can hear the whisper of God at the end.

WHAT'S IN YOUR JOURNEY BACKPACK?

Item #22: The Daily Office app. If you struggle with formulating the words for where you are in life, the Daily Office, which follows the Book of Common Prayer, has an app! Each prayer follows an ancient pattern of regular Christian devotion that is both soothing and rejuvenating.

I would give anything to have been one of those disciples that day, when Jesus physically showed up and walked beside them. But maybe I don't have to give anything to experience this. In fact, I wonder how many times Jesus joined me on my journeys, and I, like the disciples on the road to Emmaus, didn't recognize Him either.

The Bible says, "They didn't see him." This saddens me, especially because I think I would have been similarly blind to the risen Jesus. I like to think I recognize Jesus in a lot of things, but the truth is I miss Him in a lot of everyday events. This is why I continue to walk, to pray, to study, and to search so that each day I may do a better job at recognizing Jesus's presence in my life.

Brother Lawrence, who I mentioned earlier in my introduction, taught that a spiritually rich life is not so much about going out and seeking the highs; rather, it is more about opening yourself up to the realization that God is right here, right now, walking with you always and a part of every step you take.

The Road to Emmaus shows us that no matter what you think, no matter what you are not seeing or feeling, Jesus is right there, walking with you shoulder-to-shoulder, reminding you that even if you think all is lost, He has already won.

THOUGHTS TO PONDER

1. Have you ever felt the presence of God with you for no specific reason? How did it feel?
2. Do you seek out that feeling regularly?
3. What are ways that you find God in the ordinary?

Steps taken: ____________ Miles journeyed: ___________

Exercise chosen: ________________________________

Something I thought about:

____

____

____

____

Something I need to pray about:

____

____

____

____

Day

23

Paul's First Missionary Trip

For they disciplined us for a short time as seemed best to them, but he disciplines us for our good, in order that we may share his holiness. Now, discipline always seems painful rather than pleasant at the time, but later it yields the peaceful fruit of righteousness to those who have been trained by it.

—Hebrews 12:10–12

LENGTH OF PAUL'S FIRST MISSIONARY JOURNEY (FOR WHICH THE LETTER OF THE HEBREWS MAY BE ASSOCIATED): Approximately a 1,368-mile round trip

Let your determination fuel your discipline. Let your discipline fire up your search for purpose and meaning. Let your discipline create the habits for the life you want to live. But, before we get started, what *is* determination?

Determination is the emotion or neurological trigger that moves us from an inert state to an action state. It is literally that thing that drives us from point A to point B. When I wake in the morning, I am determined to have my coffee. When I dress in the morning and put on my workout clothes, I am determined to start a workout or a walk before my day begins. When I set my alarm for church on Sunday mornings, I am determined to attend church early. Determination fuels our habits, purpose, intent, and priorities. If we want certain things—not only physical things but also metaphysical, spiritual things—we need to be determined to put intent into action and make the conditions in our daily life conducive to what we want to achieve.

Discipline is not necessarily fun, but discipline helps us to create habits that fuel our intentions. And those intentions help us to start good habits and put one foot in front of another toward a specific goal.

I cannot help but reflect on Paul's determination to spread the Word of God. Paul was determined and even zealous to share God's love, His promises, and His redemptive covenant for all people. His journey is rooted in a deep and abiding love for God and for people. Every step that Paul took was driven by the determination to share this powerful love with the world. In his first missionary journey, Paul traveled from Syria, to Cyprus, to Pamphylia, to Galatia, to Cappadocia and back. Just imagine—there were no cars or airplanes to facilitate Paul's travels and take him to these faraway places. He was so determined to spread God's word that he took many of these journeys on foot, believing that God's message was more important than even himself.

I imagine that Paul, having been so profoundly transformed by his own journey on the Damascus Road, was determined to help as many people to experience the same transformation he did. Like Paul, let your determination drive your habit of practicing love in all that you do. Put love in the forefront of your thoughts. Put love in the action of your hands. Practice, practice, *practice* the art of loving in your day-to-day. It may sound easy, but if you read Paul's words and hear his story, loving God and loving people come with personal sacrifice, great discipline, and incredible determination.

Paul asked God daily to give him the determination to see his journey through. Do you ask God daily to help you with whatever you are determined to do? When I think of my habits and those things that I am determined to do, I remind myself to take a moment to pray. To ask God to be with me so that I won't falter in my journey. I ask God for the perseverance to keep at it.

WHAT'S IN YOUR JOURNEY BACKPACK?

Item #23: The Conqueror Challenges app. If you like to set tough goals and see your progress, The Conqueror Challenges app lets you sign up for various real-world distances and track your miles to the end. You'll also get a nice medal for your efforts if that's the sort of thing that motivates you!

Discipline is formed by habit. And habit is formed by repetitious behavior over and over again until that habit is a part of who we are as individuals. Practice, practice, practice that which you want to become. If you want to be more fit, more loving, more prayerful, more intentional, more mindful, more *anything,* you must establish a healthy and consistent practice.

Journeys of determination are long and hard. But journeys of determination are how God's love spread like wildfire across the nations. What are you determined to change? If you commit to it, it will become a part of who you are and change your world.

THOUGHTS TO PONDER

1. What do you want to become a part of who you are?
2. What actions do you need to take on a daily basis to make it repetitious, consistent, habit forming?
3. When and where and how long are you willing to practice this habit until it's a part of who you are?

Steps taken: ___________ Miles journeyed: ___________

Exercise chosen: ___________________________________

Something I thought about:

____

____

____

____

Something I need to pray about:

____

____

____

____

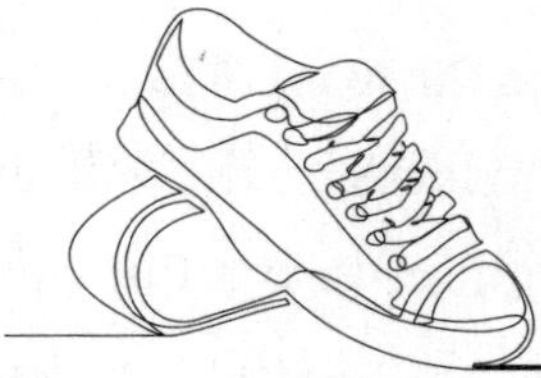

Day 24

Coming to Corinth

After this Paul left Athens and went to Corinth. There he found a Jew named Aquila, a native of Pontus, who had recently come from Italy with his wife Priscilla, because Claudius had ordered all Jews to leave Rome. . . . When Silas and Timothy arrived from Macedonia, Paul was occupied with proclaiming the word, testifying to the Jews that the Messiah was Jesus.

Crispus, the official of the synagogue, became a believer in the Lord, together with all his household; and many of the Corinthians who heard Paul became believers and were baptized. One night the Lord said to Paul in a vision, "Do not be afraid, but speak and do not be silent; for I am with you, and no one will lay a hand on you to harm you, for there are many in this city who are my people."

—Acts 18:1–2, 5, 8–10

ATHENS TO CORINTH: 54 Miles

How far would you go to spread the word of God? In our spiritual practices, it is easy to focus on the self, on our struggles, our weaknesses, and our failures. But our mission as Christians go beyond the self. According to scripture, we are called to serve others and share the Word of God with them. I don't know about you, but this part of my Christian life causes me the most discomfort. It is easy for me to write about faith and spiritual practice for those that are already believers, but it's a different story to walk the journey of Paul and share the Word of God to those who may not understand my faith.

Ever since his miraculous conversion, Paul wanted to share with the world the God who saved him, the Lord who had mercy on him, a sinner. He was desirous to spread the good news of the gospel because it was exactly that—good news!

WHAT'S IN YOUR JOURNEY BACKPACK?

Item #24: Education for Ministry. When I struggled to find my spiritual voice, one of the most profound courses I took was the Education for Ministry program at Sewanee. If you are looking for the deep dive into history, theology, reflection, and developing your call, this is a fantastic program.

It's like when you eat a delicious meal at a new restaurant or watch an amazing show that has just aired. You want to tell your friends and family all about it! But, for Paul, who had no way of easily relaying messages to others—there were no cellphones or email during Paul's time—he had to work *hard* to spread the gospel of Jesus, he had to make himself known, his voice heard, even if at times it was scary or uncomfortable.

Despite our personal reservations, we, too, are called to speak about our faith as a part of our journey. It's not something we should speak about only amongst other believers; it is something we should share with love and joy to those around us who are seeking answers themselves. Like Paul, you will likely be spurned or even spat upon. But God whispers to us to continue to speak, to seed hope, love, and faith wherever you go.

It's astounding to me that Christianity spread from Bethlehem throughout the modern world because Paul took a journey and refused to stop speaking. Imagine what God will do with you, if you refuse to stop speaking too.

THOUGHTS TO PONDER

1. Does evangelism make you uncomfortable?
2. What are ways you can share God's word that fit with who you are?
3. Are there specific places you think this is needed today?

Steps taken: __________ Miles journeyed: __________

Exercise chosen: ______________________________

Something I thought about:

____

____

____

____

Something I need to pray about:

____

____

____

____

Day
25

Preaching in Philippi

Jesus went on with his disciples to the villages of Caesarea Philippi; and on the way he asked his disciples, "Who do people say that I am?"

—Mark 8:27

BETHSAIDA TO PHILIPPI: About 32 miles

As Jesus was preaching and performing miracles in various towns throughout Israel, He was laying the foundation for our faith. After feeding four thousand hungry men, women, and children, He traveled from Bethsaida to Philippi with His disciples, cured a blind man and a deaf man, and confronting the Pharisees about their hypocrisy. When He finally arrived in Philippi, Jesus began preparing His followers for His death and resurrection and teaching them what it really means. He challenged His disciples—and us—with a profound question: "Who do people say that I am?"

Who do *you* say that Jesus is?

Think about that for a moment. It's a bit deeper than a quick response of "the Son of God." First, understanding who Jesus is means understanding why Jesus is different. It means diving into why a man dying is so profound and why

WHAT'S IN YOUR JOURNEY BACKPACK?

Item #25: Box breathing. As an "Anxious Anna," connecting to my breath keeps my feelings more stable during periods of distress. Research has demonstrated that box breathing helps calm the sympathetic nervous system, so try it out. Breethe is a great sleep and meditation app that offers breath exercises and so much more!

it should move us every day to take action. Because of Him, we have the gift of grace and can transform our brokenness into beauty.

If we believe that Jesus is the Son of God, then He is more than just man. If we believe that He suffered and took on our sins, then we believe that He is more than just God. To be both is an incredible gift. It means that God loved us so much that He was willing to experience the deep well of sorrow and pain and isolation of human existence. I feel connected to a God who cries out, "My God, My God, why have you forsaken me?" A God who can make such a vulnerable statement is a God who gets my feelings. As a feeler, I am prone to anxiety. My feelings can overtake my thoughts and sometimes make an impact on my actions. By connecting my spiritual, mental, and physical practices and realizing that God experienced all of this and more, I have become aware of God's blessings in my life.

When we say we believe, we are declaring that grace and faith are enough. We are also saying that Jesus's death was more than just the death of a man. We are declaring that in the moment of death, God has the ability to transform, resurrect, and ascend us all. For me, this is the most incredible paradox: through suffering transformation is possible. Our human existence isn't the end of the story. Through my declaration of faith that Jesus is Lord, the Messiah, the Great Shepherd, the one true God, who with the Father and the Holy Spirit are one, I am declaring that I believe. That I believe this is not the end, that God's covenant with humankind is real, and through faith, all will be made whole.

After all, faith and belief transcend the petty ups and downs of daily life. It transcends difficult diagnosis and traumas, because if I truly believe, then I have nothing to worry about. That's how I personally live with my disability. It's how I understand my cancer experience. It's how I deal with the suffering of veterans and first responders and students in my professional life. I don't believe this is the end of the story. I believe that God will fill in the cracks of my trauma and pain and mistakes and sins and all the things that have happened and make something new. God will make something good.

If I believe in Jesus, and all that the resurrection entails, then I believe that He was the one that was promised to make all things new. Including me.

THOUGHTS TO PONDER

1. Who do you say is Jesus?
2. Are you able to accept and believe that all will be made whole?
3. Do you struggle with believing that you are worthy of that gift of sacrifice?
4. Do you struggle with letting go of worry and trusting that in good and bad God can create new life and new meaning?
5. What can you do to move yourself closer to that belief?

Steps taken:___________ Miles journeyed:___________

Exercise chosen:_________________________________

Something I thought about:

____

____

____

____

Something I need to pray about:

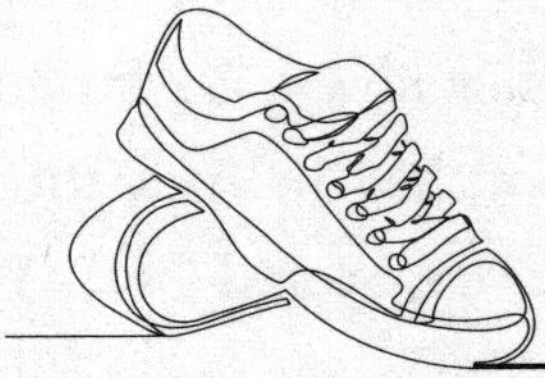

Day 26

Answering God's Call

Then Barnabas went to Tarsus to look for Saul, and when he had found him, he brought him to Antioch. So it was that for an entire year they associated with the church and taught a great many people, and it was in Antioch that the disciples were first called "Christians." At that time prophets came down from Jerusalem to Antioch.

—Acts 11:25–27

TARSUS TO ANTIOCH: 187 miles

We've been walking together now for a little over three weeks. We are more than halfway through our forty-day journey together! We've explored God's Word together, the world of the ancient Hebrews, the world of Jesus. We've explored places, ideas, feelings, concepts, and teachings that will help us grow us as Christians. It's been an incredible journey, hasn't it?

In today's passage, we learn that Barnabas and Paul continue to teach about following Jesus. We are in Antioch, where the term "Christian" was first coined, and the biblical writers record that prophets came down from Jerusalem to Antioch. I know the saying goes that all roads lead to Rome, but in the Bible, it sure seems that everything leads back to Jerusalem, where the whole concept of Christianity was born.

WHAT'S IN YOUR JOURNEY BACKPACK?

Item #26: Good socks. This one might seem a little left field, but when I wrote about Christianity chafing, I thought about how I don't like my feet to chafe on a journey. Good quality socks makes for a comfortable foot journey. You heard it from me—don't go on a journey without good socks.

But what does it make you feel like when you are called a Christian?

If I am honest, sometimes when I think about being a Christian, I squirm. Not because I am embarrassed to be a follower of Christ or am ashamed of my faith but mainly because the title weighs heavy.

I often feel unworthy to be called Christian because in every step of my journey, I struggle. Sometimes I struggle with doubt. Sometimes I struggle with authenticity. Sometimes it's with greed, or gluttony, or envy, or anger or hate. I feel all these things as a person who is fully human. The title of Christian chafes because I know that I'm not good at being a Christian on my own. And without grace and mercy, I'm not sure I could claim the title with any degree of comfort. It is only because of God's grace that I can be worthy of being called a Christian.

This week, I read about the rich man entering the kingdom of God, and Jesus's scathing remark that it would be easier for a camel to pass the eye of a needle. This passage is included in all three of the Synoptic Gospels, giving weight to the importance of the story. For that reason, it has always bothered me. By anyone's standards, I am rich: rich in love, family, friends, wealth. I have many material possessions, a beautiful house, a good job. I have many more things than I need. Because of this, I feel a weight on my shoulders as I work toward being a good Christian.

For years I would read this passage and think, there was no way I had a place in God's kingdom. I have too much. I have been given too much. I have suffered, but not enough. I have worried that no matter what kind of Christian I am, it isn't enough of the right kind of Christian. However, if you continue reading the parable of the rich man, it goes on to say, "The last will be first and the first will be last." For years, I read this as I wouldn't make it. I have come to realize, that I don't have to be first, I don't have to be perfect, I don't have to be rich or poor, but with faith, even if it's the last place, I will have a place in the kingdom of God. Because I believe. That belief is why we are called Christian.

THOUGHTS TO PONDER

1. How does the title of Christian sit with you?
2. Do you feel worthy of it?
3. Does it give you comfort, that no matter what, a place is waiting for you, even if it's the last place?

Steps taken: ____________ Miles journeyed: ____________

Exercise chosen: ____________________________________

Something I thought about:

____

____

____

____

Something I need to pray about:

____

____

____

____

Day 27

All Roads Lead to Rome

For I will not venture to speak of anything except what Christ has accomplished through me to win obedience from the Gentiles, by word and deed, by the power of signs and wonders, by the power of the Spirit of God, so that from Jerusalem and as far around as Illyricum I have fully proclaimed the good news of Christ. Thus I make it my ambition to proclaim the good news, not where Christ has already been named, so that I do not build on someone else's foundation, but as it is written, "Those who have never been told of him shall see, and those who have never heard of him shall understand."

—Romans 15:18–21

JERUSALEM TO ROME: 2,511 miles!

Paul's commitment to Christ's message and teachings took him all throughout the Middle East and Mediterranean. From Jerusalem to Crete to Malta, through the boot of Italy and north to Rome, Paul continued to preach even though he was imprisoned. I often wonder if Paul intended to go as far as Rome, or if God was working in mysterious ways. After all, it was on a prisoner ship that Paul was able to go to Rome to appeal to Caesar following his arrest for preaching. Would Christianity have spread so far had Paul not been arrested?

WHAT'S IN YOUR JOURNEY BACKPACK?

Item #27: Your favorite verse. My favorite Bible verse is Hebrews 12:1: "Run with perseverance the race that is set before us." I remind myself that when things are going tough, I need to buckle down and push hard. It also speaks to the great crowd of witnesses surrounding us, reminding me that we are never alone. What's your favorite Bible verse? Whether it's in your head or your heart, in a folded-up paper in your pocket or jotted down in your Notes app, it is certainly nice to carry with you wherever you go.

Is this again an example of God ensuring his covenant will be secured?

Over two thousand years later, Christianity is found throughout the world and in almost every country. Contrary to popular belief, Christianity is growing. We may be in a state of ebbing in the modern Western world, but God's word is alive and well and flourishing in many parts of the globe.

But this spread did not happen in a day. It didn't happen in a week. It's a race that has been ongoing for millenia. Every action, word, and prayer we take has been part of one great race to share God's beautiful covenant with all people and races.

Concurrently, the work of Christ is not done in you. If you are struggling on your mental, spiritual, or physical journey, take heart. You were not made a Christian in a day. You may have been sealed as Christ's own forever in a moment, but the work of you is something that is ongoing. It is a life's work. These habits, skills, and practices are worthy of committing yourself to being 1 percent better every day. Theologian Richard Rohr speaks to this dichotomy of Christianity, explaining that we are saved by grace alone and that faith without works is no faith. It's a process. If you could see the long view of the life you hold as Christ's own forever, you would be astounded at the ways that God is working through every moment of your life.

But to hold that long view, to build a Rome, to build a world of God's kingdom requires the discipline of an everyday life. An everyday, boring life of putting one foot in front of the other, of redirecting ourselves when we run astray or wander or get distracted. It is this initial step that helps us continue the work of God in this world. So, run with perseverance this race that God has given you. It is part of something bigger than you can see right now.

THOUGHTS TO PONDER

1. What's your life's big idea?
2. What does the long view look in your life?
3. What are ways in your everyday life you are contributing to God's kingdom?
4. What are ways you can make it 1 percent better than the day before?

Steps taken: ____________ Miles journeyed: ____________

Exercise chosen: ____________________________________

Something I thought about:

____

____

____

____

Something I need to pray about:

____

____

____

____

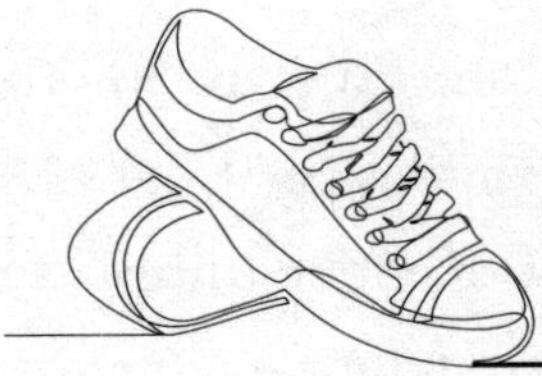

Day

28

Spreading the Word

They answered, "Cornelius, a centurion, an upright and God-fearing man, who is well spoken of by the whole Jewish nation, was directed by a holy angel to send for you to come to his house and to hear what you have to say." So Peter invited them in and gave them lodging.

The next day he got up and went with them, and some of the believers from Joppa accompanied him. The following day they came to Caesarea. Cornelius was expecting them and had called together his relatives and close friends. On Peter's arrival Cornelius met him, and falling at his feet, worshipped him. But Peter made him get up, saying, "Stand up; I am only a mortal." And as he talked with him, he went in and found that many had assembled; and he said to them, "You yourselves know that it is unlawful for a Jew to associate with or to visit a Gentile; but God has shown me that I should not call anyone profane or unclean."

—Acts 10:22–28

JOPPA TO CAESAREA: About 40–50 miles

Our desire to name things as "unclean" or "improper" or "anathema" is as strong today as it has been in years past. Human nature likes to categorize things as right or wrong, black or white. We get confused, uncomfortable, and discombobulated when issues, ideas, or actions don't fit in a neat box of our understanding. If history has taught us anything, it is that human decision-making is often flawed and deeply informed by social and cultural norms. From what I've learned from life, we need to learn and pause and make judgments through the lens of God.

In today's passage, Peter and Simon are traveling from Caesarea to Joppa to spread the word of God. Both Peter and Simon are Hebrews and are struggling with what laws apply

WHAT'S IN YOUR JOURNEY BACKPACK?

Item #28: Curiosity. Research has demonstrated that if we lean into curiosity with our perceptions about people, ideas, and things we don't agree with, we deepen our appreciation for the other person as a human. It also helps us develop a deeper understanding of nuances around certain beliefs and makes us less likely to jump to rash assumptions. Therefore, bring a curious mind with you as you walk.

to Jews, what applies to Jews that are also Christian, and what applies to the Gentiles. These conversations and discussions are forming a body of doctrine that will eventually be adopted by the later Church. But much of what is discussed are the laws of cleanliness that are a part of the Hebrew faith.

Traditionally, Peter would not have been allowed to associate with a Roman centurion like Cornelius, for he would have been deemed unclean. Through Peter, God is teaching us that the heart of righteousness is the heart that seeks God. God does not judge Cornelius for his race or cultural background but what is in his heart. For the Jews and Gentiles alike, this was revolutionary. They were being challenged to change their black and white thinking and ask themselves rather what glorifies God.

Are our thoughts ones that glorify God? Do our actions bring us closer to God? Do our judgments uphold the teachings of God? We often first fail to understand if a situation is bringing us closer to God or further away because we are quick to judge and less likely to practice discernment or understanding. And sometimes discernment takes time. It's completely acceptable to respond, if asked, that you are learning, seeking, and discerning your understanding of any issue before arbitrarily declaring something as unclean.

THOUGHTS TO PONDER

1. Do you ever feel unclean? If so, how does your perception of that shift if viewed as a child of God?
2. Have you ever considered something of the world unclean, then later changed your mind? If so, what made you change your mind and why?
3. What is something that has historically been considered unclean but today is viewed differently? Why?

Steps taken: ____________ Miles journeyed: ____________

Exercise chosen: ____________________________________

Something I thought about:

____

____

____

____

Something I need to pray about:

____

____

____

____

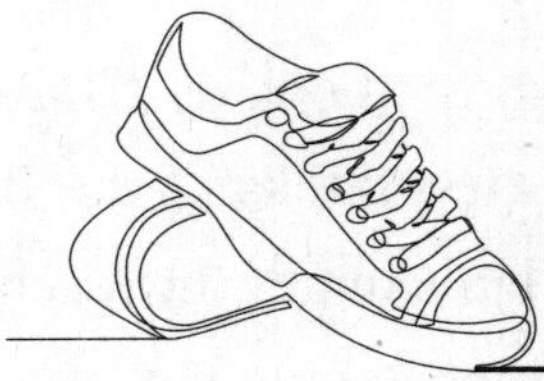

Day

29

A Voyage to Crete

Remind them to be subject to rulers and authorities, to be obedient, to be ready for every good work, to speak evil of no one, to avoid quarrelling, to be gentle, and to show every courtesy to everyone. For we ourselves were once foolish, disobedient, led astray, slaves to various passions and pleasures, passing our days in malice and envy, despicable, hating one another. But when the goodness and loving-kindness of God our Saviour appeared, he saved us, not because of any works of righteousness that we had done, but according to his mercy, through the water of rebirth and renewal by the Holy Spirit. This Spirit he poured out on us richly through Jesus Christ our Saviour, so that, having been justified by his grace, we might become heirs according to the hope of eternal life.

—Titus 3:1–7

EPHESUS TO CRETE: 617 miles

There is so much to unpack in the book of Titus considering it is one of the shortest books in the Bible. Written by one of Paul's followers, Titus shares the teachings of Paul along his own journey. It's important to note that just like Jesus, Paul had disciples spread the teachings of Christ as understanding of the Word developed. In each country/region that Paul and his followers traveled, the message was tailored to the culture of the land. It's also important to understand that the foundation of the lessons is consistent: Jesus Christ died, was resurrected, and was raised again for our sins. But each of these communities struggled with something different, and so Paul and his followers would meet the people where they were at on their spiritual journey.

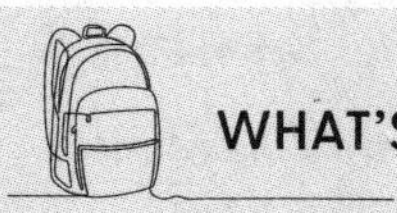

WHAT'S IN YOUR JOURNEY BACKPACK?

Item #29: Loving-kindness meditation. Loving-kindness meditation seeks to encourage Christians to center themselves on care of self, loved ones, and those that persecute them. It aims to deepen an individual's call to "love one another as I have loved you" and helps users live out their Christian call. Try loving-kindness meditation as you walk and be transformed.

According to biblical scholarship, this passage consists of the teachings spread throughout Crete, a remote island in the Aegean. As Paul traveled through the Mediterranean, the people in Crete converted to Christianity and their lives were changed forever.

This book—and this chapter specifically—is relevant to this day. First, it discusses the tension points between following rulers and following Christ. Here, Titus seems to echo Jesus's teaching to render up to Caesar what is Caesar's, but insists that our call to be patient, loving, kind, and magnanimous of spirit is not negated by following the Law. It transcends the Law. We can be obedient, lawful, and fully express our Christian spirit through our acts, even when we don't agree with the rulers or politics of those in power or around us. One of my colleagues has a phrase that I think applies here: "Assume positive intent." If we assume the best of people and respond in the spirit of love, joy, peace, and gentleness in all things, even if we disagree, then we are living out the gospel within the political and social structures we find ourselves.

Next, this chapter reminds us that everything we have is because of the grace of God. It is not our works or actions that make us righteous; it is only God's grace, love, and forgiveness. I have struggled for years to understand Paul's message in 2 Corinthians 12:9: "He said to me, 'My grace is enough for you, because power is made perfect in weakness.'" I was confused—I thought I needed to do all that I could to be perfect in God's sight. It took many years to understand that I could not be perfect, that I still sin, no matter my desire to do otherwise, that I still have weaknesses and vices and habits, despite all my healthy ways. But it is through Christ that those imperfections are made whole. It makes me fully reliant on my faith in Christ to be righteous. And I am completely humbled and have profound awe that God love us that much.

And lastly, Titus exhorts us to let go of petty arguments. As humans, we desire so fiercely to be right and justified in our choices. All three of these messages in this chapter are telling us not to be stupid. To fully rest in God's grace, whether we are right or wrong, to turn the other cheek, to assume positive intent, and to practice love, charity, grace, and gratitude. Through these practices, we get just a tiny bit closer to God on our journey.

THOUGHTS TO PONDER

1. When do you feel like you are most kind, gracious, and loving?
2. What do you think it means to assume positive intent?
3. How can you let go of stupid arguments and find peace in God's grace, not the desire to be right?

Steps taken: ____________ Miles journeyed: ____________

Exercise chosen: ________________________________

Something I thought about:

____

____

____

____

Something I need to pray about:

____

____

____

____

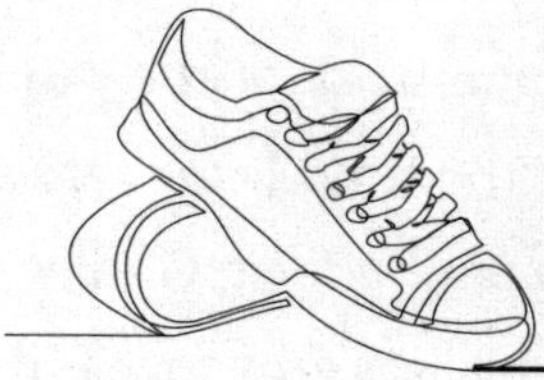

Day 30

On a Path to Wholeness

There he found a man named Aeneas, who had been bedridden for eight years, for he was paralyzed. Peter said to him, "Aeneas, Jesus Christ heals you; get up and make your bed!" And immediately he got up. And all the residents of Lydda and Sharon saw him and turned to the Lord.

—Acts 9:33–35

JERUSALEM TO LYDDA: 22 miles

The book of Acts chronicles the work of the disciples following Christ's death. By the time Peter arrives in Lydda, the Church had been built up in Judaea, Galilee, and Samaria, and the number of Christians was growing, and they were living in peace (Acts 9:31). The disciples are continuing Jesus's work of healing. They heal in Jesus's name, not through their own, and the people see the work of God through the actions of the disciples. And Peter is living the example of Christ's love on each journey he takes.

Lydda is about one day's long walk from Jerusalem. Therefore, Peter's commute to work takes a day, and then his days after are spent in healing and teaching before going to the next place. So, when Peter heals Aeneas, Aeneas gets up. And while we don't know exactly what Aeneas does to spread this gift of love, acceptance, and healing, we know that all the people of Lydda and Sharon saw him and turned to the Lord.

When people see, feel, and experience Christ's overwhelming love, forgiveness, and/or healing in their lives, they cannot help but believe. This is how the disciples spread Christianity: through love and healing.

I am humbled and blessed to have felt God's love for me in both the worst and best moments in my life. It took me many years on my journey to realize that through spiritual practices

I can cultivate a relationship with God that transcends even the highs or the lows.

Healing and belief tend to go hand in hand on spiritual journeys because it is at our moments of severe isolation, illness, fear, and despair that the *only* thing that can possibly provide hope is God. The only thing that makes sense when things don't make sense is God. And this is why you see people who have experienced the worst, often come out transformed by the trauma because they have experienced profound existential growth and understanding. I've said this before, but to me, it is not a coincidence that the cross is both a metaphor and a reality. For at the point of intersection on a cross is where transformation and suffering meet. And from that point, resurrection of a dead, hopeless, isolated person can spring.

My daily spiritual practices seek to cultivate that point of intersection because that point for me is a place of humbled joy

WHAT'S IN YOUR JOURNEY BACKPACK?

Item #30: Nature. It should go without saying that nature should be a part of your journey. However, I also want you to consider those moments you can't get out and walk or hike or run or swim when you are struggling. It can be hard. But the good news is that you can step out, for even but a moment, and breathe in the fresh air. Sometimes, just changing your scenery and taking in God's creation are all it takes for transformation.

and awe. My worst is made best through Christ. And sometimes by prayers in that place are a simple "I love you" to the one that saw something worth saving at that crossroads. Each of us hits a crossroads in our life. If you are like me, sometimes you have multiple crossroads because you must be reminded that although you are flawed, you are worthy. It's a promise that God consistently keeps to His people.

On today's walk, I encourage you simply to tell God "I love you." To let God into that place where you suffer and allow God to transform you. If you do, you will be like Aeneas, and many will believe.

THOUGHTS TO PONDER

1. How has God transformed you through suffering?
2. How do you feel when you express your love to God?
3. What do you need to feel God in that place of isolation and loneliness you experience?

Steps taken: ___________ Miles journeyed: ___________

Exercise chosen: ___________________________________

Something I thought about:

____

____

____

____

Something I need to pray about:

____

____

____

____

Part

IV

Walking with . . .

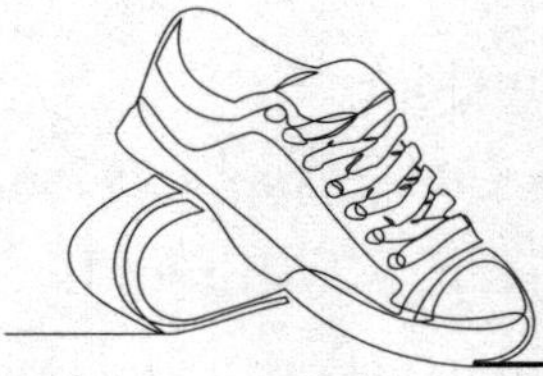

Day 31

Uncertainty

When they were few in number, of little account, and strangers in it, wandering from nation to nation, from one kingdom to another people.

When he summoned famine against the land, and broke every staff of bread.

His feet were hurt with fetters, his neck was put in a collar of iron.

For he remembered his holy promise, and Abraham, his servant. So he brought his people out with joy, his chosen ones with singing. He gave them the lands of the nations, and they took possession of the wealth of the peoples, that they might keep his statutes and observe his laws. Praise the Lord!

—Psalm 105:12–13; 16, 18, 42–45

EGYPT TO CANAAN: 5,271 miles

Lord, have mercy. Faith is a long journey.

That's how I look at this Old Testament journey of the Israelites from Egypt to Canaan. Sometimes I get exhausted just reading about it and thinking about it and praying about a journey from slavery to freedom. This is not a story where God snaps His fingers and the Israelites are magically free. There was a journey. A process. An awakening that included good and bad, ups and downs, *doubt* and understanding. Humans have this tendency to think about their experiences and sufferings as unique, but the more you study the Bible and history, you start to realize it's the same problems, different day. My mom was recently studying the books of Samuel in her Bible study group, and she came home and said, "Anna, do you know the *entire* book of Samuel is the same stuff that's going on today?"

I don't have an answer for why we don't learn from our mistakes. Why history repeats itself or why suffering, and poverty and illness are still with us. The only answer I have is that humanity is flawed. Jesus told us that the poor, oppressed, and abused would always be with us. So, we must have faith. Some of the Israelites never saw the fruition of the covenant God made with Abraham, but they persisted. They are a chosen people, and sometimes knowing you are a part of something bigger is more important than seeing the end result.

WHAT'S IN YOUR JOURNEY BACKPACK?

Item #31: Man's Search for Meaning by Viktor Frankl is one of the best books I've ever read. Take a favorite book with you on your journey or, if you prefer, use a Kindle (or a similar device or app). When you need a break, find a bench, crack it open, and be refreshed as you read.

The entire Bible is a beautiful story of God sending people, prophets, and revelations to remind us that even when we are being tested, God is there. And God doesn't just bring us out surviving; the psalmist tells us that God brings us out *rejoicing*.

I encourage you to think about your journey in different ways. Sometimes trials and tribulations are fires that we must withstand in order to be transformed into what God needs us to be for the world. We simply need to remember that we are not alone on that journey. God is always, always with us.

THOUGHTS TO PONDER

1. Reflect on your own trials and tribulations. How do they compare to the journey and experiences of the Israelites to freedom?
2. Who did God send to you when you needed help most?
3. Have you ever been sent by God when someone else needed someone on their journey?

Steps taken: ____________ Miles journeyed: ____________

Exercise chosen: ____________________________________

Something I thought about:

____

____

____

____

Something I need to pray about:

____

____

____

____

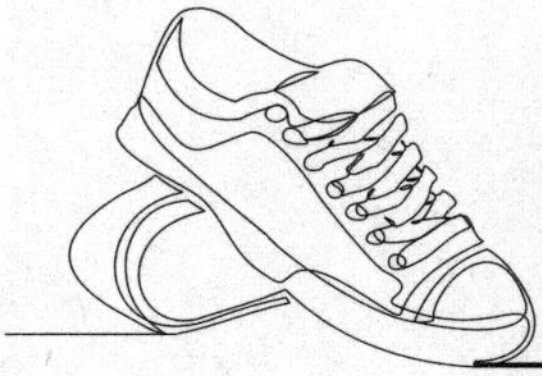

Day 32

Trauma

"For misery does not come from the earth,
nor does trouble sprout from the ground;
but human beings are born to trouble
just as sparks fly upward.

"As for me, I would seek God,
and to God I would commit my cause.
He does great things and unsearchable,
marvelous things without number.
He gives rain on the earth
and sends waters on the fields;
he sets on high those who are lowly,
and those who mourn are lifted to safety.
He frustrates the devices of the crafty,
so that their hands achieve no success.
He takes the wise in their own craftiness;
and the schemes of the wily are brought to a quick end.

They meet with darkness in the daytime,
and grope at noonday as in the night.
But he saves the needy from the sword of their mouth,
from the hand of the mighty.
So the poor have hope,
and injustice shuts its mouth."

—Job 5:6–16

ISRAEL TO THE LAND OF UZ (WHERE JOB IS FROM):
Approximately 900 miles

I cannot write about the human experience and not discuss the richness of Job's teachings. I find this personally amusing, as for so many years, Job was my least favorite book of the Bible. There was something about Job that I did not care for early in my life. I struggled to understand how he could experience so much suffering and still find joy in God.

Job did not go on so much of a physical journey, but a spiritual one. Job was a man of wealth and prosperity until life happened. He had many animals, a large and connected family, and he was recognized by his community as a righteous and good man. Satan could not believe that Job could possibly fear and honor God with all this wealth, and so he went after him. Job thus experienced one tragedy after another: the loss of all his wealth, physical assault, natural disaster, the death of all his children, illness, and feelings of abandonment by God. But through his discourse (prayer) with God, his faithfulness is revealed. The book ultimately demonstrates that righteousness is not conveyed by prosperity, and suffering is not a sign of wickedness. At its heart, the journey of Job is that faith is not a superficial experience about balance sheets and check boxes. It's about turning to God even when suffering seems never-ending.

My historical dislike of Job probably stemmed from some jealousy and shame. I wish that when I suffered, I turned to

God. Rather, I tended to turn to weeping, gnashing of teeth, and anger. There's a reason my family calls me "Drama Mama." I don't particularly like the name, but it's rather apt, and it's a reminder of the things I need to work on in myself in order to get to where Job is on his journey.

But look at the scope of Job's journey. There were times Job did not want to live. There were times Job doubted. There were times that Job was weeping and crying out and oh so angry. And yet, God saw Job as a righteous man and continued to fulfill His purpose for him. One of the best lessons I've learned from my clinical experience and education is the power of feelings. Many people fail to realize that just because we feel something, it doesn't mean that it reflects reality. In fact, in our capacity to feel negative emotions, we can often catastrophize situations and make them much worse than they are.

Sometimes I think Job got this. Although our feelings are completely normal when faced with trauma and adversity, they do not have to be the end of the story. Job's negative feelings

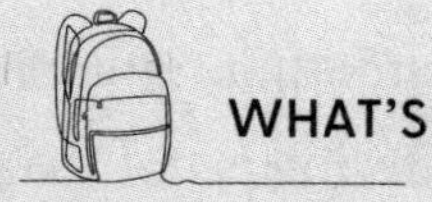

WHAT'S IN YOUR JOURNEY BACKPACK?

Item #32: *Pints with Jack* podcast. One of my favorite go-to podcasts is the *Pints with Jack* podcast which explores the teachings of author and lay theologian C. S. Lewis. If you're a big fan of Lewis's writings or theology, or if you are simply curious, I think it would be worth giving a try!

and anger were shifted as he connected spiritually with God through prayer. Yes, some of those prayers were wails, but they were still prayer. Yet again, the Bible demonstrates habits that science is validating to address suffering: prayer, stillness, meditation, mindfulness. These are the practices that bring us closer to God and help shift our negative emotions, allowing us to focus on God and what we can do, and not on what we are limited to by suffering. I mention earlier in the book, but Viktor Frankl teaches us that between stimulus (trauma) and response (feelings and behavior) is a space, and in that space is a choice and that choice is freedom (our self-agency). I would further Viktor's hypothesis: in that space of choice is God. And when we choose God, our suffering is no more.

THOUGHTS TO PONDER

1. How do you feel about Job?
2. When have you been angry or felt separated from God?
3. How did you get back to God? What were the choices on that journey that got you back?

Steps taken: ___________ Miles journeyed: ___________

Exercise chosen: ___________________________________

Something I thought about:

____

____

____

____

Something I need to pray about:

____

____

____

____

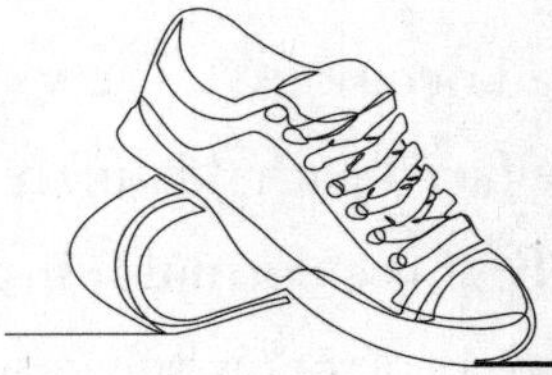

Day 33

Fear

Now the word of the Lord *came to Jonah son of Amittai, saying, "Go at once to Nineveh, that great city, and cry out against it; for their wickedness has come up before me." But Jonah set out to flee to Tarshish from the presence of the* Lord*. He went down to Joppa and found a ship going to Tarshish . . . away from the presence of the* Lord*. But the* Lord *hurled a great wind upon the sea, and such a mighty storm came upon the sea that the ship threatened to break up.*

Then they said to him, "Tell us why this calamity has come upon us. What is your occupation? Where do you come from? What is your country? And of what people are you?" "I am a Hebrew," he replied. "I worship the Lord*, the God of heaven, who made the sea and the dry land."*

—Jonah 1:1–4, 8–9

TARSHISH TO NINEVEH: 2,500 miles

Fear can make people make bad decisions.

Fear happens when we are faced with the unknown, uncertainty, traumas, and threats. Fear is a normal response, but outside of our natural instincts to protect ourselves when we are afraid, making decisions when we are afraid is rarely a good idea. Jonah's story is one of fear. He was fleeing to Tarshish and away from God's call in his life to help the people of Nineveh. The sailors in the boat reacted in fear, throwing Jonah overboard. And the people of Nineveh reacted with fear. All these instances reflect why it is crucial to seek God's direction before (re)acting, and think, discern, and pray.

Jonah's journey follows a story arc that we see in modern literature today: the hero's journey. It is one of my favorite frameworks because I am a deep fan of the struggle between good and evil, overcoming fear, and the triumph of the human spirit. In the hero's journey framework, the character sets out to explore. There is a barrier between what is known and unknown, and the individual faces challenges as he/she continues the journey into the unknown or what is feared. Every character faces the abyss. The rock bottom of their experience with the unknown until revelation occurs and a person discovers a divine capacity to survive, thrive, and grow. The individual then returns to share the wisdom learned from the journey. The hero's journey framework often mirrors life for many, and the framework provides hope.

If we were to compare this framework to the sacrament of reconciliation, we find that God has provided a similar road map for growth and hope: the individual begins the journey of life. He or she experiences sin—God feels unknown, and the individual feels abandoned and lost. The individual then recognizes the sin/fear and repents. Through divine atonement (recognition of Christ's sacrifice for your sins), the individual is redeemed, and growth and wisdom occur. The individual is called to share with others the wisdom granted from the experience of God's grace.

I like Jonah. He's not your typical hero character, but he represents the everyman experience to me. His reluctance is something that I've experienced myself. His fear of serving the Lord and what it might cost him is something with which I also sometimes wrestle. Facing and overcoming fears is a journey itself and one that we must all undergo in life. It's the fears we don't face that own us. Those fears cage us in a prison of indecision, poor health, anxiety, and isolation.

Jonah teaches us that if we first trust in the Lord (but note, Jonah had to go on a journey to gain that wisdom first), then often, all that fear and worry is unnecessary. When I was diagnosed with cancer, I was very afraid. Despite being a believer, I was afraid to die. I didn't want to leave my children or spouse. I didn't want to saddle them with a sick mom. I didn't want the pain and ordeal of living with chronic cancer. I just didn't want any of it. My fear was making me devolve. I tried to go to a behavioral health clinician, and she told me I didn't have enough faith in God. I became angry at her. Faith wasn't my issue (trust was), and I resented her words to me. But there was a grain of truth in what she was saying. I wasn't turning my fears over to God.

So, as I traversed the journey of acknowledging my fear and helplessness of my health, I realized that prayer was one of the few things that helped me face my fears. I thus decided that I would just breathe with God. I would cry with God when the pain was too much. I would share with God that I really wanted to see my kids grow up and thrive. I prayed over the knowledge and skills of my doctors. I prayed over

WHAT'S IN YOUR JOURNEY BACKPACK?

Item #33: A therapist. Although my first experience with a therapist wasn't a great one, I do have someone I go to for mental health check-ups. Finding a therapist is like finding the right shoe. Sometimes, you need to try several on to find the right fit. But it's worth it. There's no shame in needing to have a place to just talk things out. I've said before that I'm a feeler. Lots of feelings tend to sit on my shoulders, and sometimes I just need someone to talk them out. Don't be ashambed if you need that too.

each choice I made. And slowly, each step I took with God in my cancer journey was one of stronger and stronger steps.

I still ponder the remarks from that clinician who told me I didn't have faith. I still don't think that was the problem. My problem was that I was allowing my fear to control me. But that's the journey. Sometimes you have to be in the abyss, in the belly of the whale, so to speak, in order to experience the divine and come out with wisdom to share. If that's what it means to be a hero, then you are one too.

THOUGHTS TO PONDER

1. When have you been overcome with fear?
2. What were some bad decisions you made at that time?
3. How could you have leaned into your faith as a means of facing your fears?

Steps taken: ____________ Miles journeyed: ____________

Exercise chosen: ______________________________________

Something I thought about:

____

____

____

____

Something I need to pray about:

____

____

____

____

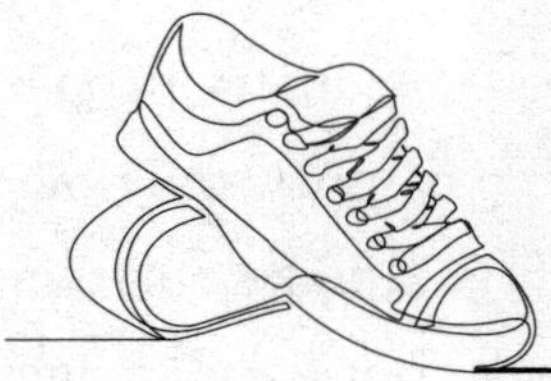

Day 34

Worry

"But if God so clothes the grass of the field, which is alive today and tomorrow is thrown into the oven, will he not much more clothe you—you of little faith? Therefore do not worry, saying, 'What will we eat?' or 'What will we drink?' or 'What will we wear?' For it is the Gentiles who strive for all these things; and indeed, your heavenly Father knows that you need all these things. But strive first for the kingdom of God and his righteousness, and all these things will be given to you as well.

"So do not worry about tomorrow, for tomorrow will bring worries of its own. Today's trouble is enough for today."

—Matthew 6:30–34

THE SEA OF GALILEE, WHERE JESUS WAS PREACHING IN MATTHEW: 64 square miles

I often struggle to see the disciples as ordinary people. My visual of them is tainted by Renaissance religious art, which portrays them as saints with gold halos surrounding their heads and old men with beards. But these images are not an accurate portrayal of the disciples, many of whom were teenagers and young adults. Some had families and jobs and all were struggling with the worries of life. I don't know if Jesus understood worry until He hung out with the disciples, who were clearly an anxious lot. But I guess that's a good thing; I think the disciples taught Jesus a lot about what it means to be human.

If I think about the amount of time I've spent worry during my life, I'm a little ashamed. In my defense, I come from a long line of worriers. Worrying is a bit of an Olympic sport in my family, as most of us often get overwhelmed with the

WHAT'S IN YOUR JOURNEY BACKPACK?

Item #34: *The Chosen. The Chosen* is a TV show that imagines the lives of the disciples during the time of Jesus. I think it really helped me see the disciples as humans, as ordinary individuals called by God for an extraordinary mission. If you're walking on a treadmill, this is a great show to watch on your phone or tablet.

"what-ifs" and anxiety. In my defense, I've been working on crushing this habit. I'm slightly less anxious today than I was ten years ago, but it's an ongoing process.

If I equated the time in my life spent in worry to miles on my life journey, I wouldn't be surprised if a good third to half of those miles were from worry. This disappoints me. Worry makes you walk round and round in circles and doesn't really get you anywhere. It takes a lot of work but ultimately yields very little progress in the goals you want to achieve.

I love the book of Matthew. It's full of so much good instruction on living a good life. In this parable, Jesus is telling us, just stop with the worry. God's got it.

My mother-in-law tells me that if I was really praying about my worry, I'd give it to God and not take it back. She's got a point (don't tell her!), but my response is often that God knows I worry, and this is an ongoing process in my life. I am very bad about giving the worry to God and walking away. Somehow, worry tends to come find me. And then I must go through the process of letting my worry go again. I've told my mother-in-law that God's used to me at this point in my life, and I am grateful that God is patient, God is constant, and God is forgiving. It means that even though I know my worry is for naught, if I pray about it, there will be a place for those worries, no matter how many times they come back.

THOUGHTS TO PONDER

1. Where do you fall on the worry spectrum?
2. Does praying help you manage your worry?
3. How much time do you think you've wasted worrying in your lifetime?

Steps taken: ___________ Miles journeyed: ___________

Exercise chosen: ___________________________________

Something I thought about:

____

____

____

____

Something I need to pray about:

____

____

____

____

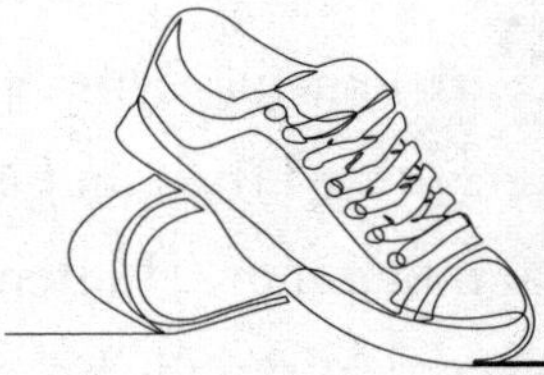

Day

35

The Unknown

When he was sitting on the Mount of Olives, the disciples came to him privately, saying, "Tell us, when will this be, and what will be the sign of your coming and of the end of the age?" Jesus answered them, "Beware that no one leads you astray. For many will come in my name, saying, 'I am the Messiah!' and they will lead many astray. And you will hear of wars and rumors of wars; see that you are not alarmed; for this must take place, but the end is not yet. For nation will rise against nation, and kingdom against kingdom, and there will be famines and earthquakes in various places: all this is but the beginning of the birth pangs."

—Mathew 24:3–8

THE MOUNT OF OLIVES: 2,493 feet

In October 2014, I was diagnosed with follicular lymphoma. It brought a screeching halt to everything I thought I knew about life, God, faith, health, and so much more. I often feel that, at the time, I was psychologically and spiritually hijacked. I was stuck and paralyzed and deeply afraid. The future was uncertain, and I didn't know how to deal with uncertainty. I've already shared that I am a worrier at heart. Well, I also dislike change. I am a creature of habit. And I like to be in control. Cancer takes all that away from you.

As I write this reflection today, I have cleared another year of being in remission (yeah, me!). It's always with mixed feelings that this day comes. I am humbled and grateful for another year. I grieve for those that are going through their

WHAT'S IN YOUR JOURNEY BACKPACK?

Item #35: Sticky notes. I often write reminders to myself when I want to remember the wisdom God has taught me on my journey. Right now, a sticky note on my computer says, "One thing at a time." Send yourself messages—whether it's on a Post-it or a Notes app—that remind you what you know to be true. When worry and uncertainty crop up, you'll be reminded that you've faced this before and can make it through again.

own journey. And I am forced to reflect on the past ten years and where I am today. It reminds me of the hurt and loss I felt, and it's easy to get pulled into the mire of those feelings.

In this passage, Jesus has climbed the Mount of Olives to be with His disciples. They were beginning to realize that Jesus wasn't going to be with them forever. Things were going to change, but they weren't sure what life would be like. Jesus was presenting them with a lot of uncertainty and asking them to walk by faith.

When you've had your life hijacked by something major, it requires that same faith to receive the information, trust in doctors, God, friends, family, and others, and put one foot in front of another to get to the end place, postcancer (or other tragedy). When struggling with disease, trauma, or any kind of suffering, we are called to walk with a lot of faith because we don't necessarily know what the end will entail. The hardest thing I had to accept with my cancer diagnosis was that I might not live. None of us are promised tomorrow in the physical sense, but in the spiritual sense, God has promised us so much more. I had to realize that even if my cancer journey didn't go the way I wanted, God would care for my family and be with them, while I was hopefully rejoicing with the saints.

Some journeys are incredibly long, scary, and uncertain. When we focus those feelings into a prayer to God and continue to put one foot in front of another, we also will find God at the end of our journeys, no matter how difficult that journey may be.

THOUGHTS TO PONDER

1. Are you on, or have you been on, a long or uncertain journey?
2. What was it?
3. What were the complex feelings you had to experience?
4. Where did you find God in that journey?

Steps taken: ____________ Miles journeyed: ____________

Exercise chosen: ____________________________________

Something I thought about:

____

____

____

____

Something I need to pray about:

____

____

____

____

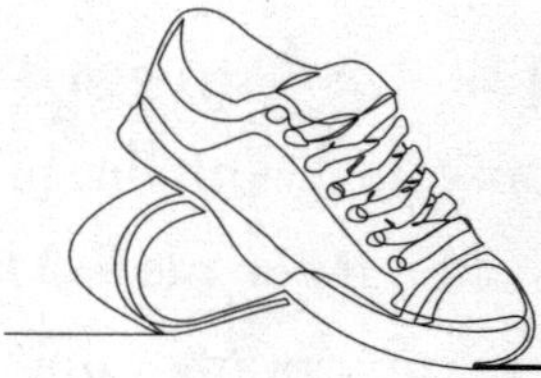

Day 36

Doubt

As he walked along, he saw a man blind from birth. His disciples asked him, "Rabbi, who sinned, this man or his parents, that he was born blind?" Jesus answered, "Neither this man nor his parents sinned; he was born blind so that God's works might be revealed in him. We must work the works of him who sent me while it is day; night is coming when no one can work. As long as I am in the world, I am the light of the world." When he had said this, he spat on the ground and made mud with the saliva and spread the mud on the man's eyes, saying to him, "Go, wash in the pool of Siloam" (which means Sent). Then he went and washed and came back able to see.

—John 9:1–7

THE POOL OF SILOAM: 225 feet long.

As a person with a disability, I've always struggled with the passages in the Bible about others with disabilities and Jesus's healing. These passages often make me feel like I don't have enough faith. There's a portion of my mind that feels like if I only believed more, then maybe the magic wand would give me back my hearing and my health. I envy the man at the Pool of Siloam.

But Jesus also says that God is working through people in their infirmities. They—and I—are not sick because of sin, nor a lack of faith, but for a bigger purpose that we cannot see. That bigger purpose gives me hope and meaning and a great deal of joy. When I am frustrated by my disability, I remind myself that this loss also brought a gift that I did not have before: compassion, empathy, faith, and perseverance, all fruits of the spirit.

WHAT'S IN YOUR JOURNEY BACKPACK?

Item #36: Baptismal water. I often dip my finger in the baptismal font before communion to cross myself. It's a lovely reminder of the personal covenant between me and God. Keep a vial with you as you walk or hike. Having a bit of holy water is always spiritually uplifting.

This passage also mentions the disbelief of the man's neighbors, who could not believe he was healed. They couldn't quite fathom that Jesus could make miracles happen. Similarly, in our day and age, many people doubt that those who are suffering and have experienced trauma can possibly experience joy and peace.

The current social media crisis continues to teach young people that the perfect image, the perfect filter, the perfect home, décor, job, etc., is one's goal in life. Our messaging to society today focuses on getting "likes" for a social persona that does little to prepare individuals for when things go wrong. It is no surprise to me that mental health is considered a "public health crisis," as rates for depression, anxiety, suicide, and alcohol and drug abuse continue to soar. We've abandoned our worth as children of God with fruits of the spirit in exchange for superficial likes.

The man at the pool "journeys" into the Pool of Siloam to wash after Jesus paints mud over his eyes. Two hundred and twenty-five feet isn't an exceptionally long journey, but it is profoundly symbolic to wade into the "mud" of your experience and have it washed off into new life, new possibilities, and new promises. Our baptism does the same for us.

Many people have gone through great loss and come out the other side shining. They experience a spiritual baptism that reflect the joy and peace that only God can provide. They too are provided with gifts of the spirit that change the hearts of those who doubt each day.

THOUGHTS TO PONDER

1. Does your face and soul shine with the light of God, reflecting the joy in your life outside the sorrow?
2. How are ways that you do this?
3. What made you believe in your journey that God was with you?
4. How can you share that with others?

Steps taken:__________ Miles journeyed:__________

Exercise chosen:____________________

Something I thought about:

____

____

____

____

Something I need to pray about:

____

____

____

____

Day 37

Anxiety

Then he told them a parable: "Look at the fig tree and all the trees; as soon as they sprout leaves you can see for yourselves and know that summer is already near. So also, when you see these things taking place, you know that the kingdom of God is near. Truly I tell you, this generation will not pass away until all things have taken place. Heaven and earth will pass away, but my words will not pass away."

—Luke 21:29–33

THE SEA OF GALILEE: 33 miles (in circumference)

Before I die, I'd like to walk the perimeter of the Sea of Galilee. Jesus shared most of His profound teachings around this lake, and I cannot help but think that those waters are holy. I imagine the hills, soil, and trees being permeated by His presence as He stood on the sea's shores. I imagine stepping in those waters and stepping back into time and seeing Jesus face-to-face.

For many, death brings on anxiety. We profess to believe that Christ will raise us from the dead, but it's difficult for our human brains, so preoccupied with logic and reasoning, to believe it sometimes. But I do believe it's true.

When I was diagnosed with cancer and told my lymphoma was noncurable, I got faced with the reality of my potential death. At thirty-eight, I wasn't prepared to say goodbye to my children or husband. Heck, I like my life! I love Jesus, but

WHAT'S IN YOUR JOURNEY BACKPACK?

Item #37: A large water bottle. Water is the gift of life. And hydration is incredibly important to your physical well-being. It's refreshing, cleansing, and restoring. It's also not surprising to me that Jesus baptizes with water. We need it with us every day.

man, I wasn't ready. I know I have spoken about it before, but there was a lot of anxiety and feelings going on at that time of my life.

Having been in remission now for ten years and counting, I'm still not ready to die. But my perspective on death has changed since then. As I grappled with the process of living with cancer as a part of my story, I recognized that all life ends at some point. And if I truly believe that Jesus comes to raise believers from the dead and that there is so much more to life than just live, pay taxes, and die, then I also believe that God is a part of this whole process. I ultimately came to understand that should I die, (a) my body would be made whole and that my suffering would end; and (b) while it would be hard for my family, God would be with them through the process of letting me go.

I'm still not ready to die, but now it doesn't scare me as much. I think where the switch flipped for me was the realization that it is a lot easier to believe that God would be with me and my family in death than live with the anxiety and fear and worry of what life would be like if I died. I remind myself of this outside of my cancer. As my children launch into life and become independent and go off without my husband, it's easy to become anxious. So, I pray daily that God keeps them safe.

In this passage from the Bible, we are told that we don't know the hour that Jesus will return, but we should be prepared. I think our journeys in life are all about preparing us for that moment when we die. Revelations would tell us that it will be the profound, singular moment when all the believers at once will go to heaven. But I've always wondered if that moment was individual. You see, none of us know when we'll die, but I believe that in that moment, Jesus is there. We don't know the hour, but He will be there.

THOUGHTS TO PONDER

1. How do you feel about dying?
2. Does it make you comfortable/uncomfortable to know that Jesus will be with you in the end, no matter what?
3. What do you think about the journey in the afterlife?

Steps taken: ____________ Miles journeyed: ____________

Exercise chosen: ____________________________________

Something I thought about:

____

____

____

____

Something I need to pray about:

____

____

____

____

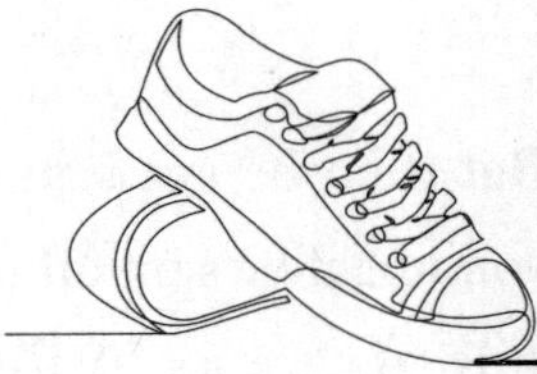

Day 38

Faith

He said, "Come." So Peter got out of the boat, started walking on the water, and came towards Jesus. But when he noticed the strong wind, he became frightened, and beginning to sink, he cried out, "Lord, save me!" Jesus immediately reached out his hand and caught him, saying to him, "You of little faith, why did you doubt?"

—Matthew 14:29–31

LAKE GENNESARET: 4 miles long, 2 miles wide

Jesus said, "Come."

So, Peter came to Him. But then he got scared. I know this Peter. He's the one who wonders if he's bit off more than he could chew. He's got a family to care for. A fishing business. Taxes to pay. He's got other fish to fry, and while following Jesus is awesome, it's also a little scary sometimes.

Have you heard Jesus's call in your life and hesitated? Have you looked with squinty eyes, suspicion, or fear? I know I have. My response is usually along the lines of, "What could you possibly need *me* for?" Then, I wonder what the personal cost will be, what I will have to sacrifice if I answer Jesus's call. Other times, I simply feel lazy. But Jesus consistently whispers, "Come."

And when I obey, when I lead into faith, I never regret it. I don't know why at this point in my life that I still question Jesus's call on me, but I do. I guess it's because I still can't quite believe that even with all my baggage, sins, and brokenness, Jesus could possibly have a job for me. And yet, Jesus whispers, "Come."

In my day job, I work in health and wellness. I've worked with soldiers, first responders, healthcare workers, and students. I've always believed that organizations are well when they are led from a place of wellness. One of my charges to my team is that it's never a wrong decision to be a good human.

And they have taken this guidance to heart. When we meet, we start our meetings with check-ins, voicing our gratitude, discussing their opportunities to be a good human, as well as administrative stuff. It's a framework that works well for us. And I am humbled to get to lead in this way.

But part of leading is doing what we believe. There's an individual in our organization with whom I have butted heads. We have fundamental disagreements in what's important strategically, and I question whether we have similar values. I usually avoid this person when I am able. However, I had noticed this person was not looking well. And my Spidey Sense was going off. Jesus was whispering "come" and calling me to reach out to this individual. I didn't want to go because I really don't like this person.

But then I recalled how Jesus often calls us to the unlovable, the unlikeable, and those with whom we disagree. And I was reminded that even though it was going to make me uncomfortable, it was never a wrong decision to be a good human. So, I reached out. I'm not sure where it will go from here, but I answered that call in a very mundane, daily call of "come" that Jesus whispered.

Jesus is doing that in your life as well. In all the troubled spots, dangerous seas, everyday and difficult journeys, he's whispering, coaching, cheering, and calling. In my devotional time today, I was reading from Billy Graham's *Unto the Hills.* In today's reflection, Graham describes a passage from Ephesians 3:10: "God's purpose is now to show the rulers

WHAT'S IN YOUR JOURNEY BACKPACK?

Item #38: An apple. The work of faith is hard work. Healthy fuel keeps me going for that next time that Jesus says, "Come."

and powers in the heavens the many different varieties of his wisdom through the church" and describes this teaching in the infinite, omniscient, and omnipresent capacity of our God to simply *know.* If we believe in all aspects of our God, then to have faith in all things means leaning into Jesus's call to us. I believe that God has seen the vastness of our potential and purpose in our life and when we lean toward that call to come, then we come closer to everything that we can possibly be.

Sometimes the hardest part of our journeys is taking that step of faith. Trusting in the unknown. Trusting in that call from God to come. Because we often think far less of ourselves than God does. I want you to know that you aren't alone in those feelings. And as a recovering questioner, I struggle with trust, to let go and let God. But when you do take a risk and trust in God, you won't be disappointed.

THOUGHTS TO PONDER

1. Have you heard Jesus say "come" in your life?
2. What was it about?
3. How did it make you feel?
4. How did you lean in or away from that call?

Steps taken: ___________ Miles journeyed: ___________

Exercise chosen: ___________________________________

Something I thought about:

____

____

____

____

Something I need to pray about:

____

____

____

____

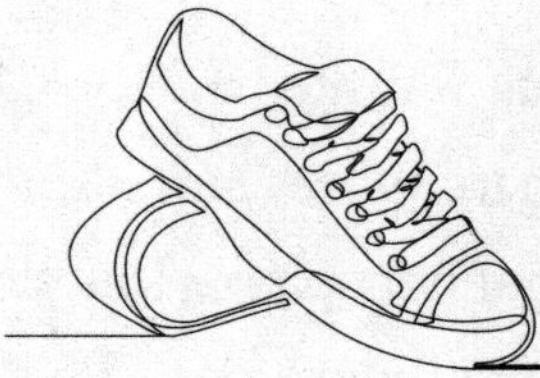

Day 39

Revelation

To him who loves us and freed us from our sins by his blood, and made us to be a kingdom, priests serving his God and Father, to him be glory and dominion for ever and ever. Amen.

Look! He is coming with the clouds;
every eye will see him,
even those who pierced him;
and on his account all the tribes of the earth will wail.

So it is to be. Amen.

"I am the Alpha and the Omega," says the Lord God, who is and who was and who is to come, the Almighty.

Revelation 1:5–8

ISLAND OF PATMOS: 7.5 miles long

I knew when I started this book that I wanted to write about John on Patmos. I have been there twice, and it's a holy experience. There is something about holy places that brings the reality of the Bible to life in the modern day. This was my experience in the Cave of the Apocalypse on the island of Patmos in Greece.

According to tradition, Saint John was exiled to the island of Patmos by the Roman emperor Domitian, who was persecuting early Christians. The Romans considered prophecy to be a form of magic and astrology that threatened political power and order. Consequently, John's writings were considered a threat and punished by banishment.

But although John was imprisoned, his spiritual life flourished. His is another story about the transformative, redemptive

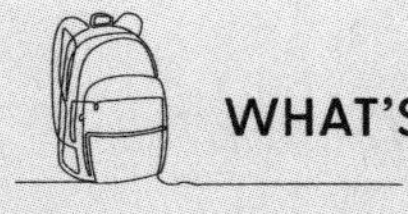

WHAT'S IN YOUR JOURNEY BACKPACK?

Item #39: The Creeds. I pray the Creeds during my workout warm-up. I like that they are a part of my fitness routine, as they allow me to reaffirm my beliefs as I exercise. There's something important about digging into the minutia of what you believe about your faith. Writing your own Creed can be a way for you to connect to those details of faith and lean into other areas you need to explore.

power of God's grace in the middle of suffering. And through this suffering, wisdom was revealed about the future. This is Revelation.

I've never liked Revelation. It's gobbledygook to me. It makes me squirm because my logical brain struggles with much of the content. I must really, really study this book to get beyond my initial response, to fully appreciate the joy John is describing in seeing the covenant God has made with His people realized. John reveals to us that we don't need to be afraid.

Revelation to me is not about an end. It's about a promise. It's about God as the Alpha, the Omega, the beginning, and the end, and that there is so much more than this life that we currently lead. When I lean into Revelation, I begin to understand why the Church says, "With angels and archangels, and with all the company of heaven, we proclaim God's name."

God has made a promise. All our time together has been exploring God's promises throughout history, and His consistent, constant love, commitment, and care for people is evident if we study God's word. My practices reveal to me that I want God in my heart, my mind, and in my words. I am a better person for practicing being the kind of person God thinks I can be. I am happier, and despite all that's happened in my life, the brokenness of my body, I am made whole.

When I journey with Revelation, I journey with confusion and discomfort, but also awe, joy, humility, purpose, promise, and hope. There is so much more being written about God's story, and I want to be a part of it.

THOUGHTS TO PONDER

1. How do you really feel about the book of Revelation?
2. Is there a way you can lean into the book that helps reveal the nature of God on your own journey?
3. Are there parts of Revelation that give you hope for the future? What are they?

Steps taken: ___________ Miles journeyed: ___________

Exercise chosen: ___________________________________

Something I thought about:

____

____

____

____

Something I need to pray about:

____

____

____

____

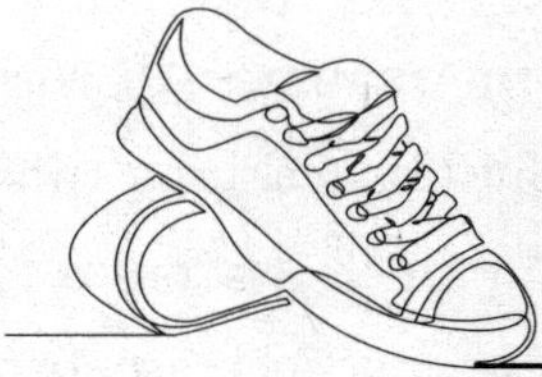

Day 40

Wisdom

For wisdom is more mobile than any motion;
because of her pureness she pervades and penetrates all things.
For she is a breath of the power of God,
and a pure emanation of the glory of the Almighty;
therefore nothing defiled gains entrance into her.
For she is a reflection of eternal light,
a spotless mirror of the working of God,
and an image of his goodness.
Although she is but one, she can do all things,
and while remaining in herself, she renews all things;
in every generation she passes into holy souls
and makes them friends of God, and prophets;
for God loves nothing so much as the person who lives with wisdom.

—Wisdom of Solomon 7:24–28

DISTANCE TRAVELED: ***Infinite.*** The journey with God never ends.

Aeschylus is attributed with the saying, "All wisdom comes through suffering." But this teaching can also be found in Ecclesiastes 1:18: "For in much wisdom is much vexation, and those who increase knowledge increase sorrow." I have found that my wisdom was derived not just through suffering, but also being exposed to trauma, facing it, being exposed to it again, and then realizing that I had the wisdom to face it.

In this final passage from the Bible, I was struck by the similarities in the description of wisdom as to my thoughts about the Holy Spirit. To me, that means wisdom is there in us always, for the Holy Spirit dwells within us (1 Corinthians 6:19–20). The Spirit teaches us about the covenant of God with God's people. The Spirit teaches us about Jesus's sacrifice of love for who we are, despite our sins. The Spirit opens us

WHAT'S IN MY JOURNEY BACKPACK?

Item #40: YOU! I always think about my readers on my walk because I want to remember those that have been with me in my writing journeys. By sharing my words, we get to experience God together. And there's no better walk than one with companions.

to the promise of redemption and wholeness through repentance. The Spirit feeds our developing wisdom through our experiences. And as we nourish that relationship with God, it's not just through suffering that wisdom develops, it becomes a part of our process of everyday life.

This book is about a journey with God. God is with us each day on our journey. Sometimes we feel very close to God—often in the moments of extreme despair! Sometimes we feel that God is absent from that journey (also, sometimes in the moments of extreme despair!). But if God is omnipresent—God is there. If God is the Holy Spirit, then God is there. If Jesus died, rose, and will come again, then God is there in that covenant, in that promise that God has made to God's people.

In every step you took on this journey with me, God has been there. In every step you will take in the future, God will be there. This book has been about how we reflect on all the journeys in the Bible, and how God was there. Through our practices (mind, body, and spirit), I hope you've been awakened to God's presence in your life.

God is there.

THOUGHTS TO PONDER

1. Where do you think you have gained most of your wisdom?
2. How do you think about God as a part of this wisdom?
3. How can you continue to nurture your relationship with God on your daily walk?

Steps taken: ___________ Miles journeyed: ___________

Exercise chosen: ______________________________

Something I thought about:

____

____

____

____

Something I need to pray about:

____

____

____

____

Afterword

Hallelujah! It is finished!

My journey to completing this book was a four-year journey that included a global pandemic, the loss of my father and my dog, two job changes, a retirement, a child going to college, a spouse retiring, and so much more. There were highs and lows and everything in between. There were lots of steps and miles and a couple of injuries and illnesses. There were also many times I wasn't sure I had it in me to write another book and yet here we are. There were times I didn't feel like writing and times I didn't feel like walking, but I did so. This book is a book about journeys, and I'm hoping that it has inspired you to go on some of your own.

As you read each entry and respond to the prompts at the end, my prayer is that you learn something about yourself and God that you didn't know before. More than anything, I hope you are grateful for the time we spent together. I know I am!

I am grateful for God. I wish I could express more profoundly how this journey has led me closer and closer to Him.

I've discovered within myself this deep awe that leaves me humbled and thankful and fills all the cracks of my brokenness and makes me whole. I am grateful for my husband, whom this book is dedicated to. Each year that we walk our journey together, I am humbled he's by my side. I am grateful for my kids, who think their mom is both weird and cool. Although they don't quite understand all my experiences, they love me anyway, and I'm grateful for getting to experience motherhood because of them. I'm grateful for my editor, who pushes me to write better and go deeper than I sometimes desire but always leaves my work better than where it started. And readers, I'm grateful for you.

For those of you who are young on your spiritual journey, take heart. Your love and awe of God will only grow and grow and grow. Sometimes, you will be baffled, confused, and afraid, but always, always, always God will be faithful and will lead you on a better journey than you could imagine for yourself. You just can't always see it in the middle of each step you are taking. Just keep walking!

For those of you who are more seasoned on your journey, I hope this book has helped you deepen your own growth toward God. My time with my readers is something I cherish. I always say that every word written is worth it if it helps just one person. I challenge you to do the same and share your story with others.

Humans are made for community. And journeys, while sometimes solo, are often better when we share them with others. So, walk together. Love God. Love each other. And keep walking.

With Love and Blessings,
Anna